DOCTOR-PATIENT RELATIONSHIP IN AFRICA

From the Institute for Medical Psychology of the Albert Ludwig University of Freiburg i. Br.

DOCTOR-PATIENT RELATIONSHIP IN AFRICA

Second Edition, 2026

INAUGURAL-DISSERTATION

For the attainment of the degree of Doctor of Medicine of the Medical Faculty of the Albert Ludwig University Freiburg i. Br.

Submitted in: 1983
Dean: Prof. Dr. med. W. Bredt
1st Reviewer: Prof. Dr. med. S. Goeppert
2nd Reviewer: Prof. Dr. med. J. Cremerius
Date of Doctoral Degree Award: April 14, 1983 "Magna Cum Laude"

FILIPE DOM MASQUIL

Printed in the United States of America.

ISBN-13: Paperback 979-8-9966899-0-3
ISBN-13: Hardcover 979-8-9966899-1-0

Library of Congress Control Number: Pending

DEDICATION

Omnia mea mecum porto, "I carry everything I need with me."

Dedicated to my mother: She was the first to show me how beautiful and meaningful listening and smiling, laughing and crying can be for human relationships as well as means of communication.

CONTENTS

ACKNOWLEDGMENTS

My special thanks go to Prof. Dr. med. Sebastian Goeppert, who allowed me to write my thesis under his supervision. I would also like to thank his colleague, Dr. Gottfried Fischer, Academic Councilor, who, together with Prof. Goeppert, generously supported me during my work. I would like to thank Mrs. Elke Schleeh for her excellent work as a secretary, for her support, and for her friendship.

I would also like to express my gratitude to Prof. Dr. med. Diesfeld and his colleagues, Dr. med. habil. Dorothea Sich, Dr. med. habil. Axel Kroeger, and Dr. Pflederer from the Tropical Institute in Heidelberg. I was able to have a conversation with them before starting my dissertation and received some interesting literature suggestions. The conversation was recommended and arranged by Prof. Dr. med. Eduard Seidler. I am grateful for his kindness.

Dr. Dagmar Wagner-Robertz encouraged me with her great interest in the work and supported me with some literature suggestions. My heartfelt thanks to her as well. I would like to thank Dr. George Specht and the Caritas Association for their support and friendship. I also want to express my thanks to Dr. M. Krim, who generously supported me before I received a scholarship.

I met many friends during my studies who made life in Freiburg enjoyable. I am thinking, for example, of the Hans Glunkler family, but also of many others whom I unfortunately cannot name individually here. My heartfelt thanks go to all of them as well.

Last but not least, I would like to thank the Otto Benecke Foundation for granting me a scholarship. My special thanks go to Dr. Bauer and his colleagues.

PREFACE

The doctor-patient relationship is, among other things, a personal confrontation between doctor and patient.

I would like to introduce myself and my country to the reader. This preface, so to speak, reflects my own connection to the subject at hand.

I was born in Mozambique as the eldest of five siblings. My father was the youngest of ten siblings. This was a favorable situation for my father, as he had less responsibility for the family and was able to pursue adventures, such as coming into contact with Western civilization. In our home, the older brothers had to look after the younger ones, and the younger brothers were raised from a young age to treat their older brothers with love and respect.

This custom exists almost everywhere in Africa, particularly in families organized as patrilineal extended families. "As soon as the mother stops breastfeeding the child (at the age of 3 to 4 years), the child is entrusted to the care of an ascending hierarchy of siblings, playmates, and relatives (including the parents themselves)."[i]

At the age of 18, my father found a job as a **Muleque** (servant) in a Portuguese family. His tasks included looking after the children, doing housework such as cleaning, making beds, shopping for groceries, helping in the kitchen, and so on. In return, he received "free meals" and money, which he could use to buy trousers, shirts, or sweets.

One time, my father WITNESSED an accident: WHERE ANOTHER MULEQUE dropped a pot of food belonging to his employer. The woman, who was nearby at the time, became so furious that she slapped HIM.

In my tribe, physical punishment is very restrained. Children are generally not beaten, and if they must be punished, certain rules apply. A mother is not allowed to physically discipline her son if he is older than 12, and a father cannot discipline his daughter if she is older than 12. When physical punishment occurs, it is meant as a warning or a sign that the child must obey the parents, and the parents must not show anger during the act. Woe to the father or mother who is caught by their in-laws or grandparents striking a child.

When the Portuguese saw that Africans did not beat their children, they interpreted it as if they were not disciplining them. For this reason, they implemented systematic physical punishment as part of the "civilization" of the natives: "*A palmatoria e o cavalo marinho*"[ii]

My father had been with the Portuguese family for only two months and had not yet fully absorbed the wonders of civilization or the life of the city (Beira). He was not convinced that it made sense to stay any longer. He was simply horrified to have been struck by a woman at his age. His own mother would never have dared to do such a thing! He was not only affected but also deeply insulted, humiliated, and shocked!

Without saying goodbye, he ran back to his village, to his "Ndau tribe."[iii] Had this incident never occurred, perhaps my father would have stayed in the city of Beira and might have been corrupted, as part of the colonization of Africa involved the introduction of "liquor."[iv] Mozambique was no exception, especially with the addition of Portugal's renowned wines.

In truth, this "incident" turned out to be a *felix culpa-a* "blessing in disguise."

Now my father was back with his tribe, back with the **Mashikiri** (Portuguese: Masquil), a great tree that has always "protected" our tribe from misfortune. My father told this story about Beira to me and all my siblings. He told us that since then, it had been his sacred wish that none of his children, no matter what, should ever find themselves in such a situation namely, being struck by a Portuguese man or woman.

In any case, since my father was the youngest child, he had a great sense of security, knowing that all his siblings would not abandon him. As I mentioned earlier, in our tradition, the eldest siblings are obligated to care for the younger ones, both spiritually and/or materially.

Now back in his tribe, his interest in tradition was fully awakened, and he approached it with great intention. I also benefited from this, and the passion with which my father spoke about our tribe and traditions has fascinated me to this day.

This also explains why, despite my long stay abroad, I remain deeply rooted in tradition.

At the beginning, I thought that school, and later my studies, would transform me into a new person, allowing me to see everything in a different light. Since everything unfamiliar is alluring, and because I believed that education would change me, I tried to explore various things.

"The Portuguese divided all Africans into two groups: assimilated and indigenous, civilized and uncivilized. The census book laid down certain rules which had to be followed before one could obtain passage to the civilized' status: the applicant had to speak Portuguese, show proof in his behavior and dress that he had rejected his African past; finally, he had to have a profession or employment."

Thus, the conflict for my father grew stronger. He believed that as long as he told us children the history of our culture faithfully, we would keep it in our hearts. This would then be compatible with our integration into Portuguese society. He thought a good start would be for me to be baptized.

Well, as a child, I stood before the priest with my parents. The priest asked, "Name?" The answer was, "Oom!" It was not allowed; I needed to have a holy name, as is customary in the Catholic Church. Through the priest's quick decision, I came home as Filipe. Oom was allowed to remain on my birth certificate, but only as a second name - Filipe Oom. On the same day, my father was baptized as well; his name was also Filipe. It was a great day for our family with a new holy name.

My parents now had to live two different lives. One life was that we wore shoes and the same fashion as the Portuguese, and the other life was that they maintained close relationships with relatives who had not taken any steps toward civilization. As a result, we also had to participate in all the rituals of our tribe. For this "other life," my father had a second house built in the village so that we could spend weekends and holidays there. Otherwise, we were "good" Portuguese citizens and only spoke Portuguese in public. These "two" lives were experienced by most assimilated people. In one example, Azevedo tells of an "Assimilado" who finds himself in conflict:

"Bento's personal life was not simple. In many ways, he was still tied to the African values of his parents and his compounds. This caused conflict in planning his

future. He was happy in his life with Juha, but he often sat quietly in his mud and straw house at the end of the day and recalled the teachings of his elders: young Mozambicans are told that they must have many children in order to carry on the family name and to support the wide family."

Personally, I liked the stories and rituals of my tribe. The conflict became conscious only when I fell ill. I felt very bad and was taken to the hospital, where I had to stay for observation. In the company where my father worked, there was a company doctor for both the Portuguese and the staff. The nurse was a good friend of my father's, one of those who had fled to Zimbabwe with him. Often, when I was ill, I was taken to the hospital. The doctor came, examined me, and I received the medication. Meanwhile, my father had arranged with the nurse that the traditional healer could visit me at night. He then came with my parents and other relatives, performed his ceremony, and I also received his medicine. The medicine from the doctor was bitter, most likely quinine, and the medicine from the traditional healer was sweet: an extract of roots in a tea with sugar. I preferred the medicine from the healer.

When I lived in the boarding school of a mission school, the difference between a doctor and a traditional healer became clearer to me. The focus of the lessons was religion, and among other things, the healer was portrayed as pagan. After some time, when I returned home, I began to voice objections to the healer, just as I had heard in school.

My father's explanation was: "We are Christians. I know what the missionaries say, but there is a difference between African - Christians they now live in two realities. One is the reality of our ancestors, which will continue to protect us as long as we uphold our traditions, and the other is that Jesus helps us when we pray to him. Actually, things are even better for us now, not just one, but two."

I would like to point out here that this attitude towards tradition and Western views is ubiquitous among Africans. Even Albert Schweitzer made the following remark about his patients: "The 'elders' pour schnapps into the water and tobacco leaves to appease the evil spirits, so they will allow the fish to be caught and do no harm to anyone. When these ceremonies were stopped a few years ago, an old woman got tangled in a net and drowned." "But most of you are Christians," I remarked, "you don't believe in these things." "Of course," he replied, "but anyone who would speak against it or even smile while the spirits are being offered tobacco and schnapps, sooner or later, would find themselves poisoned. The fetish priests do not forgive. They live among us, without being known."

As I said, this was a similar attitude of my father toward tradition, even though we were Christians. I must also admit: I found the traditional healer very sympathetic; his dance, his singing were a lot of fun for me. It was simply wonderful to watch him sweat, so much so that I often forgot I was sick. All his efforts were so impressive that I hardly doubted him when he promised me and my family that I would soon be healthy. I often did recover; and if not, I could also go to the doctor, or visit both at the same time.

When I left the country, I thought those were "the good old days," and now I am in Europe, where traditional medicine and witch doctors are regarded as insignificant. Even from Africans in Europe, I would expect them to be free from what is called superstition. But four months ago, my conviction was put into question. I went to Berlin to visit my Mozambican acquaintances. There was also a girl from Nigeria with us. After she left, I asked my acquaintance why she looked so distressed. He told me that she was friends with a doctor from Nigeria. But here, she met another man and wrote to her old friend about it. She suggested breaking off the friendship with him. The young doctor replied, saying that his grandfather was a healer, and he had protected him and his family. Within a year, she would have to pay for her decision. Something tragic happened to her in Germany. In fact, after receiving her Nigerian friend's response, she had recently undergone surgery for colon cancer.

Before I continue with the story, the reader may wonder how a traditional healer can also cause illnesses. I will report on this point later (probably in Chapter III). But perhaps for now, it is enough to point out once again that Albert Schweitzer, in Lambarene, asked himself the same question when he observed how his patients viewed him:

"My name among the natives in the Galoa language is 'Oganga,' which means fetish doctor. They have no other word for doctor because the black healers are all simultaneously fetish doctors. My patients logically assume that the one who heals illness also has the power to cause it, even from a distance. The thought of being regarded as both a good and simultaneously dangerous being is strange to me." What have I tried to show? The examples mentioned in the preface are meant to be no more than a few case studies. I want to bring to light the details, the feelings behind the conflicts.

There are also other reasons why I have included examples from home. A comprehensive, scientifically written book about Mozambique, along with statistical data, describes the situation at the time remarkably well. However, the author came to a wrong conclusion.

"In September 1958, Dr. Ralph von Gersdorff undertook a research trip to Mozambique to broadly describe the political, economic, social, and cultural conditions in Mozambique." Prior to this, he had undertaken study trips to Pakistan, Portuguese India (Goa), and Ceylon. "Since 1956, he had worked as an advisor for development areas (country studies at the Hamburg World Economic Archive) and made study trips to Africa in 1957 on its behalf." So, a scholar with experience in field research. The following is an excerpt from Dr. Gersdorff's book:

Population

Mozambique was the first Portuguese overseas province in which a census was conducted. The "civilized" population was counted for the first time in 1928, and the "non-civilized" in 1930. "Civilized" population (Law No. 36 of 12.11.1927) refers to all individuals with white, brown, or yellow skin, as well as mixed-race people and those Black people who speak Portuguese, have adopted the Christian religion, show good conduct in military service, live an European lifestyle, and have sufficient property or income to support their family, whether as an independent farmer producing for the market or employed by an employer. They are therefore full citizens of the Portuguese Republic, but also have corresponding duties, such as paying various taxes (depending on profession) instead of the low head tax for non-civilized people and covering medical costs, which they would not otherwise have to pay. Many non-civilized individuals simply do not choose to become full citizens for material reasons, even though they meet the above criteria. The number of Black people regarded as civilized was 4,554 in 1955. Racial discrimination is officially prohibited but occurs everywhere.

The basic law for the overseas provinces of 1930 (incorporated into the constitution in 1951) states: "It is one of the most important tasks of the Portuguese nation to fulfill its historical mission by possessing and colonizing overseas territories and civilizing the native population living there, influencing them with its culture, a function which was transferred to it according to the 'Padroado Portugues do Oriente." Marriages between whites and blacks are rare; due to the influence of white women, they automatically led to exclusion from society. The number of mixed-race individuals is decreasing. While white women on average have two children, people of color have about four children.

An estimate of the population before 1908 was only made in 1900. It amounted to 735,152 inhabitants, of which 3,014 were white, 1,436 mixed-race, and 730,702 black. For 1908, the total population was

1,477,460, for 1917 it was 3,652,008, for 1920 it was 3,028,761, for 1923 it was 3,530,377, and for 1926 it was 3,523,611. Since 1930, the "civilized" population has been counted every 5 years and the "non-civilized" population every 10 years.

Payment of civilized:	1928	1935	1940	1945	1950	1955
Total:	35,570	45,750	55,451	60,115	91,954	117,405
White:	17,842	23,131	27,438	31,221	48,213	65,798
Yellow:	896	1,056	1,449	1,565	1,613	1,945
Indians:	8,475	8,304	9,147	9,700	12,630	15,235
Mulattos:	8,357	13,259	15,641	15,784	25,149	29,873
Blacks:	-	-	1,776	1,845	4,349	4,554

In 1950, those mulattos who did not live in the European style were also counted as "civilized." This accounts for the significant increase in the number of this group. The number of foreigners steadily decreased. In 1928, they made up 28.9% (10,278 people) of the civilized population, in 1935 it was 17.6% (8,073), in 1945 it was 12.8% (7,686), in 1950 it was 8.4% (7,748), and in 1955 it was 5.6% (6,694). Nevertheless, Mozambique (also due to many tourists and transit traffic from neighboring countries) has more international character than, for example, Angola. The largest foreign colony is that of the Indians from the Indian Union. For the year 1955, the following numbers are recorded:

Indians	12,343 people
Pakistanis	1,579 people
English	879 people
Chinese:	769 people
South Africans	450 people
Italians	360 people
Greeks	308 people
Germans	306 people
Swiss	155 people
Dutch	121 people

Among the last two groups, there are many missionaries. Dual citizens are only counted as Portuguese nationals.

109,707 people were counted as Portuguese full citizens, including:

- 63,386 White
- 29,586 Mulattos
- 11,044 Brown people from Portuguese India
- 4,538 Black people
- 1,153 Yellow people from Macau.

The majority of the "civilized" population comes from Mozambique itself (50.6% in 1950), 35% are from mainland Portugal, 8.4% from abroad, and 5.4% from other Portuguese overseas provinces. Among the White population, the Portuguese from mainland Portugal were the most numerous (66% in 1950, 32,134 people); most came from Lisbon, Porto, Guarda, and Viseu.

The districts with the largest "civilized" population in 1955, as in previous censuses, were Lourenço Marques, Manica e Sofala, Mozambique, and Zambezia. The two largest cities, Lourenço Marques and Beira, had a "civilized" population of 44,032 and 16,668 people, respectively. Due to improvements in transportation infrastructure and the development of agricultural exports, there was a decrease in the concentration of the White population in Lourenço Marques in 1955, and a larger occupation of the interior of the country: from 1950 to 1955, it increased by only 26.5% in the Lourenço Marques district, while in the Gaza district, it grew by 119.8%, in Inhambane by 35.9%, in Manica e Sofala by 51.1%, in Zambezia by 56.9%, in Mozambique by 60.4%, in Cabo Delgado by 38%, and in Niassa by 52%.

The previous counts of the "uncivilized" population resulted in the following numbers:

- 1930: 3,960,261
- 1940: 5,030,179
- 1950: 5,646,957

The largest population in 1950 was in the Mozambique (1,309,999 people) and Zambezia (1,156,244 people) districts. The most densely populated (including the "civilized" population) districts were Lourenço Marques, with 19 people per square kilometer, Mozambique with 16, Zambezia with 11, and Inhambane with 8. The other districts had a density ranging from 2 (Niassa) to 7 (Gaza) people per square kilometer.

For the entire territory and population, the population density in 1950 was 7.4 and is estimated to be 8 in 1955.

In 1950, a total population of 5,738,911 people was counted, of which 91,954 were "civilized" and 5,646,957 were "uncivilized." By 1955, the "civilized" population had increased to 117,405. Assuming that the "uncivilized" population grew at the same rate from 1950 to 1955 as it did from 1940 to 1950, it would have reached 6,094,000 people by 1955. Together with the "civilized" population, this results in a total population of 6,211,405.

In 1950, 156,380 "uncivilized" individuals were working in the South African Union and in Rhodesia, while 16,744 were counted as coming from the neighboring areas of Mozambique.

Each year, about 3,000 to 4,000 Portuguese from mainland Portugal immigrate to Mozambique (4,021 in 1955, with 505 returnees), while very few foreigners (97) and Portuguese citizens from other overseas territories (60) come to the country. This is due to the restrictive government policy. Many Goans work as civil servants, lawyers, and doctors, while those from the Indian Union are almost exclusively active in trade.

From the quote, it can be inferred that the Portuguese sought to make the indigenous people full citizens, which meant that the natives had to abandon their culture in favor of the Portuguese way of life. However, this only led to tensions and frustration. What people, who are occupied by another power and forced to abandon their culture, will not suffer conflicts as a result? Nevertheless, Dr. Gersdorff concluded the following at the time:

"Conflicts like those in Kenya, cannot arise in Portuguese East Africa because the black population has enough fertile land for cultivation. The government guarantees its ownership and the land it occupies. They are not displaced by incoming whites. White immigrants are settled on land equipped with irrigation systems; but blacks are also given settlement plots there."

However, Mozambique waged a longer and more radical liberation war than Kenya.

I hope that with the example of my father, I have not given the reader the impression that I am attempting to write a novel, but rather that I have aimed to illustrate, through concrete examples, the feelings and contradictions that were awakened by the Portuguese colonial state and its goals.

The reader may wonder what the connection is between my lengthy discussion of the political situation in Mozambique and the topic at hand. The connection is intentional. I believe that it is not enough to only learn about the various characteristics of a country, but also to understand the attitude and expectations of the population towards the doctor and their reactions. Only then can the doctor gain an overview and, as a result, treat patients more effectively.

In Mozambique, as in many African countries, health policy was an expression of political and cultural oppression. Accordingly, the population also felt exploited and used in the healthcare system. The population of Mozambique and the current government (FRELIMO) asked, after independence, what significance Western medicine had. At that time, it served the power of the colonial state, and even though it benefited a few indigenous people, it was only because they were kept healthy enough to continue working for the colonial masters. The following quotes will show the attitude the government of Mozambique has taken regarding healthcare as a reaction. In an official document from the Ministry of Health, the following can be read:

"Slave owners, large landowners, merchants, patricians, free men, feudal lords, bourgeois, capitalists all the rich and privileged are 'treated' at home by doctors who are generally at their exclusive service, and whose prestige and wealth prove the respect of their clients. The slaves, the small peasants or poor artisans, the serfs, the proletarians, all the miserable people, are either not treated, or are treated by other doctors, or through a different type of care given out of necessity to preserve their working strength or to satisfy the demands of social struggles. They must resort to special institutions or collective hospices, reserved for centuries for the exploited classes, the marginalized. It is from here that hospitals will arise.

The bourgeoisie did not go to the hospital for treatment (and only in private rooms, special infirmaries, or private clinics) until the degree of differentiation in technical and scientific diagnostic and treatment methods reached a level that required its organization in hospital institutions, a special source of prestige for the doctors practicing and leading them.

After the French Revolution, and especially from the beginning of the last century, as industrial and scientific development progressed, medicine began to have more precise scientific knowledge and to dominate increasingly sophisticated techniques for treating diseases.

The medical profession acquires a clearly mercantile character, with all its components: a commodity that is sold the healthcare services, the seller the medical profession, and the buyer the public.

Thus, the character of the 'liberal,' 'independent,' 'private,' and 'lucrative' profession emerges, placed in the service of the bourgeoisie. This type of medicine is, moreover, the ideological emanation of the interests of the bourgeoisie."

... In this context, in capitalist societies, the medical schools and university hospitals play a decisive role in the perpetuation of this state of affairs. In fact, it is here that students are taught the spirit of elitism; it is here that the idea of the individual 'doctor-patient' relationship is disseminated as the supreme goal, with the patient placing themselves in the hands of the doctor, who becomes the sole judge.

The interference of this type of medicine in the health of the community is practically nonexistent, but the truth cannot be revealed, as this would mean the ruin of the entire system. It is therefore necessary to instill in the medical student-apprentice exploiter (merchant of medicine)- the 'academic' mentality, the supreme form of elitist thinking.

Under these conditions, medicine becomes a 'RELIGION,' medical schools and university hospitals transform into 'PLACES OF WORSHIP,' and the 'Professors' become the 'CLERGY.'

Even when the practice of private medicine is forbidden to 'Professors of Medicine' (as is the case in many industrialized capitalist countries), they cease to be direct exploiters, but remain a category of personnel paid by the system, often rewarded by large multinational corporations, to perpetuate the system."

This is a harsh attitude towards the doctor. I would like to remind once again that I have already suggested that this is a reaction, even a hyperallergic reaction, to colonialism and its health policies. A rage against 500 years of exploitation and injustice. Nevertheless, one should keep the "great goal" in mind and recognize that this reaction can be a path for the development of a just healthcare system. The reaction is also there to ask us we doctors in Mozambique what kind of doctors we will be. Will we be like those from the colonial era?

The answer is expressed by how we shape our relationship with our patients and our country.

I believe I am touching upon an important point about African doctors abroad. From the quote, it can be inferred that the government is generally hostile towards doctors, so one might feel unwelcome.

Matomora K. S. Matomora from Tanzania also shows in his dissertation that the colonial infrastructure and the colonial healthcare system pursued the same goal.

"1884/85 saw the formal partition of Africa by the European powers in Berlin. The era of direct colonization broke in. The champions of colonialism and imperialism of the day expressed their aims of colonizing Africa with unsurpassable clarity. Cecil Rhodes, after whom Rhodesia (Zimbabwe) was named, had the following to say:

"I was in the East-End of London and attended a meeting of the unemployed. I listened to wild speeches, which were just a cry for 'bread, bread,' and on my way home I pondered over the scene and became more than ever convinced of the importance of imperialism. My cherished, idea is the solution for the social problem, i.e. in order to save the inhabitants of the United Kingdom from a bloody class struggle, we colonial statesmen must acquire new lands to settle the surplus working-class population. We must find new lands from which we can easily obtain raw materials and at the same time exploit the cheap slave labor that is available from the natives of the colonies. The colonies would also provide a dumping ground for the surplus goods produced in our factories. The Empire, as I have always said, is a bread-and-butter question. If we want to avoid class struggle in the United Kingdom, we must become imperialists."

Tanzania was to come under German rule....

a) The German medical personnel came to serve the colonial troops, who were conducting their most feared military expeditions to enforce unconditional subjugation and destroy any resistance to their rule of power. Indeed, as Clyde himself notes, the doctors were themselves actively involved, while "carrying a first aid box in one hand and a pistol in the other...."

The official colonial policy even as late as 1935 was to reserve the manning of high posts and training to the British: "Admission to the unified colonial medical service is necessarily confined, broadly speaking, to persons of British nationality... It is the policy to train the local inhabitants for minor posts in the health service."[v]

I would stray too far from the topic if I were to describe how the healthcare system in Tanzania is organized. Nevertheless, it is my conviction that African doctors must reflect on the philosophy of their country and its healthcare system. It is not enough for a country to take a series of measures; our involvement is also crucial. But for this, we need an overview of the whole system. Otherwise, we would move from one system to another, from one *coup d'etat* to the next, losing everything painstakingly built each time, resulting in confusion about the future.

That many missteps have been taken in the attempt to industrialize Africa does not need to be proven through World Bank statistics or UN reports. We ourselves admit it. For example, in the fall of 1980, African literature was the focus of the Frankfurt Book Fair. There, African writers highlighted, as a central theme, the misguided technological development with misplaced priorities, which led to the destruction of the values of our familiar traditions. For instance, Nkem Nkwanko (Nigeria), in "*My Mercedes is Bigger than Yours,*" as commented by Al Imfeld, "his book becomes almost allegorical for all of Africa... Entirely in the tradition of a comedy, such a hollow life cannot offer much. The Mercedes ends up in a ditch, and the hero in the grave."

We cannot afford to repeat the same mistakes in healthcare policy as were made during Africa's industrialization. This would lead us to an even worse situation. It is already regrettable that we still suffer from so many infectious diseases. Should we also import so-called diseases of civilization before we have dealt with our own illnesses?

Further Reading

1. Mario Azevedo, ***The Returning Hunter***, ibid., p. 9
2. Paul Parin, ***The Contradiction in the Subject***, ibid., p. 159
3. Mario Azevedo, ***The Returning Hunter***, ibid., p. 32
4. Mario Azevedo, ***The Returning Hunter***, ibid., p. 46
5. Albert Schweitzer, ***Self-Testimonies***, ibid., p. 107
6. Albert Schweitzer, ***Self-Testimonies***, ibid., p. 95
7. Ralph von Gersdorff, ***Mozambique,*** Publications of the German Africa Society, in: The Countries of Africa, Volume 14, Bonn, Schroeder, 1958, p. 7
8. Ibid.
9. Ralph von Gersdorff, ***Mozambique***, ibid., pp. 15 ff
10. Ralph von Gersdorff, ***Mozambique***, ibid., p. 7
11. ***Primary Health Care in Mozambique***, People's Republic of Mozambique, Ministry of Health, 1977, pp. 21 ff
12. See also Al Imfeld, African Literature in: ***My Mercedes Is Bigger Than Yours***, Wuppertal, Peter Hammer Verlag, 1979, p. 5

Papal commission to the Portuguese Crown for the mission and the appointment of priests in the Orient.

Notes

[i] Paul Parin, ***The Contradiction in the Subject: Ethnopsychoanalytic Studies***, Frankfurt/M., Syndikat: 1978, p. 144.

[ii] Mario Azevedo, ***The Returning Hunter***, USA: Interculture Associates, 1978, p. 9.

A palmatoria: a punishing device made out of wood, shaped and sized like a human hand. Its surface has several holes designed to draw the flesh from the hands of the punished.

Cavalo marinho: a long rope made from hippopotamus skin.

[iii] Ndau ("Lion's People"): a tribe that is part of the Bantu people, present in both Mozambique and Zimbabwe.

[iv] Albert Schweitzer, ***Self-Testimonies***, Munich, C.H. Beck Verlag, 1967, p.86:

...On the riverbank, abandoned and dilapidated huts. "When I came to this country twenty years ago," said a merchant next to me, "these were all thriving villages."

"Why are they no longer thriving?" I asked. He shrugged and replied quietly, "Liquor."

See also pp. 168-169.

[v] Matomora K.S. Matomora, ***The Development of the Infrastructure in Medical and Health Care Service in Tunduru District***, Tanzania since 1965, Heidelberg University: Dissertation, 1979, pp. 16 ff

INTRODUCTION

The Thesis

A doctor-patient relationship in Africa is only possible if the doctor can successfully interpret the patient's "unique" experiential world within their own frame of reference, beginning with the anamnesis or conversation. This then leads to mutual respect, which is the *conditio sine qua non* for maintaining a relationship. Only under these circumstances can the doctor fulfill their task of education effectively. Without a good doctor-patient relationship, most prevention and health measures in Africa will be met with rejection by the population.

The Problem

The perception of illness (etiology, pathophysiology, and therapy) in African culture differs significantly from that of Western medicine at least at first glance. From experience, when people from different cultures come into contact, this often triggers insecurity, defense mechanisms, and even contempt for the other culture.

As long as this contempt exists (whether consciously or unconsciously), genuine help cannot be provided, nor can a favorable environment for mutual understanding be created. The same applies in medicine: a doctor cannot establish a relationship with a patient if they do not understand them. However, the path to this necessary mutual understanding unfolds in stages, with mutual respect being the pinnacle. Only then can the doctor truly help the patient, and the path to education becomes clear.

The traditional healer, who has always stood by the African's side (despite being outlawed during colonial times and even after independence in some African countries), could perhaps reveal the "secrets" of their success in building relationships with African patients to the doctor. On the other hand, the close collaboration between the African patient and the traditional healer can lead both parties into a dilemma: the contempt directed toward the traditional healer could "per continuum" spread to their patients.

For this reason, the traditional healer was sometimes regarded as a symbol of so-called superstition and identified or even incorporated into traditional African culture. This raises a valid question: who, exactly, is the traditional healer?

But behind this question lies the most important aspect of this work: what are the positive and negative aspects of the mindset or worldview of the African patient regarding illness and health, and how can the doctor come to understand them? In other words, is it possible to find an analogy between this "unique" experiential world of the African and Western medicine, so that a doctor can interpret the patient's frame of reference? Throughout this work, I will highlight such "foreign" situations and concepts and attempt to explain them in light of Western medicine, and vice versa. This is not to merge the two systems they remain distinct but to search for a common ground that can serve as a basis for the doctor-patient relationship.

As the foundation for building this relationship, the "client centered" therapy approach by Rogers is proposed. This is not only because this theory is already familiar to doctors but also because it "shares many similarities with the 'conversation' of the traditional healer," which is familiar to the African patient. Concrete examples will be provided and explained using this model.

This is a theoretical work based on data from renowned field researchers of the African scene. My title, *Doctor-Patient Relationship in Africa*, should not be viewed as an attempt to generalize about the entirety of Africa. Nonetheless, I have included quotations from the literature that have universal validity and are also familiar to me from my own cultural background.

The following quotes support this idea:

"The broadest category encompasses all African cultures. One seeks cultural traits that can be considered characteristic of Africa and that distinguish it from other cultural 'continents': the West, India, China, Islam, etc. If one finds more commonalities among the various African cultures than between African and other cultures, it becomes increasingly justified to group them into a single category.

L. Frobenius identifies these commonalities as 'the African,' while L. S. Senghor and the writers associated with the journal *Presence Africaine* attempt to capture it in the concept of 'Negritude.' J. Jahn refers to it as the 'agisymbiotic culture,' reviving a term used by Ptolemy on his world map for all regions south of Libya. These efforts place great emphasis on the intellectual aspects of a culture: philosophy, myths, artistic forms, and symbols. These elements are undoubtedly significant, but they are not the only ones. If one wishes to discover the 'essence of Africa,' it is interesting to compare it to what lies outside of it."[vi]

Or as Kwame Nkrumah, former President of Ghana (1957-1966), expressed in his book *Africa Must Unite*:

"We have developed cultural differences that shape our attitudes. All of this is the inevitable consequence of our history. Despite everything, I am convinced that the forces that favor unity are far stronger than those that divide us. Every time I meet Africans from different parts of the continent, I am pleased to see how much we have in common. It is not just our colonial past or shared goals; the commonality runs much deeper. I can best describe it as a feeling of oneness, a sense that we are all Africans."[vii]

To this truth, I would like to add another, equally valid truth: there is also a "feeling of oneness" with all humanity, and we can learn from one another. As brothers in a large family the human race we can support each other toward the same goals: happiness, peace, and health.

"People are the children of humanity of all times, all zones, whether they dwell under birch trees or live beneath palm fronds.

Whether they bow before the Christian God or before Wodan, Whether they shelter in rags, or adorn themselves with purple."[viii]

I hope that this work can therefore serve as an impetus for the doctor-patient relationship, not only in Africa but more generally.

Further Reading

1. Len Holdstock, ***Indigenous Healing and the Person-Centered Approach of Carl Rogers***, in: Curare, Journal for Ethnomedicine and Transcultural Psychiatry, Vol. 4, 1981, pp. 31-46.

Notes

[vi] Jacques Maquet and Herbert Ganslmann, ***Africa, the Black Civilizations***, Munich, Kindler Verlag, 1970, p. 14.

[vii] Joachim R. Klicker, ***Africa***, Frankfurt/M., Peter Hammer Verlag, 1979, p. 128.

[viii] Verses from Weber's Dreizehlinder, cited in ***Psychology of the African Student***, by Abbe Dr. Ntetem - unpublished.

CHAPTER I

THE UNIQUENESS OF THE MEDICAL HISTORY IN OUR CULTURE

1. The danger of misinterpreting the medical history of the African patient by the doctor

Doctor: "What brings you to me?"

Patient: "My aunt was with me last week, and when she left, she looked at me strangely, and since then I've had this stomach pain."

Doctor: "When does this occur, mostly before or after meals?"

Patient: "Every time my child says something, or when I think of my aunt, I notice... etc."

My reaction as a doctor trained in the West:

"Please tell me, where does it hurt?" And as a result:

a) The doctor may lose the trust of the patient.
b) The doctor might arrive at a "psychologically oriented diagnosis" because he interprets the patient's world differently.
c) Prematurely targeted questions may hinder the patient's trusting account of the illness progression.

The following medical histories are genuine examples from field research by A. B. Chilivumbo and are used to illustrate this particularity.

Patient A

Questioner: How are you?

Patient: A little better.

Q.: What are you suffering from?

P.: I was employed at a certain place, and while working there, some of my fellow workers practiced magic with the intention of getting me out of work. One day, as I was going home, I met a strange figure on the way and passed by it. When I reached home, I began to suffer from various illnesses.

Q.: How do you feel now?

P.: There is a slight improvement.

Patient B

Q.: What are you suffering from, madam?

P.: I feel piercing pains here and there all over my body.

Q.: When did you come here?

P.: Three weeks ago.

Q.: So how do you feel now? How do you think you got the disease? Do you perhaps think it's from some bad people?

P.: I don't know whether it's from God or not.

Q.: Is your home nearby?

P.: My home is in Mulanje (100 miles from Mwanza).

Q.: How did you come here?

P.: I came by bus.

Patient C

Q.: How are you, madam?

P.: Not so well.

Q.: Where do you come from?

P.: I come from Zomba (100 miles from Mwanza).

Q.: When did you come here?

P.: I came on Wednesday.

Q.: What is wrong with you?

P.: I have heart troubles.

Q.: How does it trouble you?

P.: I feel burning pains in my chest, which makes me not feel well.

Q.: For how long have you had this trouble?

P.: This is the ninth year.

"The reported illnesses carry mystical aspects. In the patient's mind, the illnesses are more than somatic, and Bwanali represents a mysterious healer-one with extraordinary talents. In his cure, medicinal potency is shrouded in mystical influence. It operates on two levels: the biochemical process and the psyche. The method is both curative and preventive. It aims at physical cure, puts the patient's anxieties at ease, reinstates in the patient the will to live, frees him from fear, and restores him to normal functioning within the social fabric."

The above-mentioned complaints are not uncommon in Africa. Some serious African researchers found this type of medical history so foreign that they arrived at incorrect interpretations and conclusions. There are many examples in the literature, and I would like to briefly report on a book I studied with great interest. It is called The Search for Security, An Ethnopsychiatric Study of Rural Ghana, by M. J. Field. Many complaints and medical histories are astonishingly well described, and they seemed very familiar to me. However, when the author made his diagnosis or drew his conclusions, I disagreed with automatically be classified under various psychiatric disorders. It is truly insufficient for a doctor to list all the basic and accessory symptoms according to E. Bleuler or first-rank symptoms according to Schneider, and other secondary symptoms, in order to arrive at the definitive diagnosis of "schizophrenia" etc.

I ask for understanding: I do not mean that there is no schizophrenia, endogenous depression, etc. in our society. There are mentally ill people everywhere, even in Africa. I only want to emphasize that the response, the confrontation, and the interpretation of illnesses can be different when compared to the West, and that the doctor is tempted to categorize many symptoms or complaints under the diagnostic categories of Clinical Psychiatry. My example at the beginning of this chapter could lead a doctor, who asks targeted questions to the woman, to prematurely diagnose the psycho-vegetative exhaustion syndrome or a disguised depression.

A possible approach in the case of suspected mental illness is suggested by Field himself: "But on the whole, Africans are shrewd at diagnosing madness and often know the main differential diagnosis - epilepsy, mental defect ("not clever"), trypanosomiasis, and "spirit-possession". On several occasions when they declared a patient to be 'becoming mad,' I first disagreed with them, but later found that they were right" with Clinical Psychiatry, I would like to add another quote: "In general, however, specialists hold the view that the term for our so-called mental illnesses, insofar as they are not of organic origin, are so culturally specific that any comparison with primitive forms remains highly questionable".

2. Examples of the Importance of a Good Doctor-Patient Relationship for the Medical History, Diagnosis, Therapy, and Patient Compliance

Already in the first clinical semester, we learn: "At the beginning of the path to diagnosis, complaints (medical history in the first sense) and findings are essential.

Table 5. Reported Reasons for Non-Attendance TB. Clinic Ncihana

Reasons for non-attendance	1st semester 1969	2nd semester 1969	1st semester 1970	Total
Away from home for family affairs	13	27	18	58
Away for work	3	-	-	3
Passed away at home	3	2	2	7
Poor performance status	5	13	14	32
Assaulted	2	1	-	3
Sickness at home	2	14	11	27
Under treatment of herbalist	2	7	1	10
Mother in puerperium	1	-	1	2
Mother under treatment	2	10	7	19
Trivial excuses	5	14	12	31
No excuses	11	4	16	31
Total	49	92	82	223
Number of different patients visited	38	71	69	178

The medical history serves to provide you with information about complaints and previous diseases, enabling you to make a diagnosis. It also gives your insight into the patient's personality, allows you to establish a trustful relationship with the patient, which is often crucial for effective therapy, and it provides the patient with a welcome opportunity to express themselves, in a sense, as a catharsis" (Gross).

In other words, the diagnosis supposes a good medical history, which in turn requires a good doctor-patient relationship, and the latter is a prerequisite for effective therapy and patient compliance. This fact should deepen in our awareness during and after our training and should be mastered.

When I told Prof. Dr. H. Diesfeld, the director of the Medical Tropical Institute in Heidelberg, about my plan to write this paper, he said to me: "This relationship is not only lacking in your country or in Africa, but it is also imperfect here. In the Federal Republic of Germany, our doctors talk too little with the patients; they focus more on lab results, CT scans, and other technical devices."

This remark impressed me even more when I visited a long-time German acquaintance. I asked him where he and his family had been. After a pause, he told me: "I am ashamed of this, but this is what happened. I went to a conference in Hamburg, and my wife went with the children to her parents' place. There, I noticed that I had either lost or left my wallet at home. I was also very tired, and I had slept poorly for the past three nights. So, I went to the conference organizer and asked if there was a place where I could sleep and borrow money, since I didn't have my wallet with me. Later, the organizer brought a man who then looked at me closely and recommended that I go to the hospital. Despite my claim that I wasn't ill, 20 minutes later, an ambulance arrived and took me to the psychiatric ward. I was immediately given haloperidol, which I had to swallow in front of the nurse. After the ward doctor got my address, he called my wife and told her that I was suffering from a severe psychosis. I felt very hurt when I realized that my wife automatically accepted the doctor's diagnosis." He then continued, telling me that he could hardly sleep in the hospital because other patients were screaming and running around all night, and how he was shaking and couldn't walk properly.

He presented me with a classic case of Parkinsonism. After receiving money from his wife, he escaped from the hospital. Later, he discussed with a lawyer the possibility of suing for unlawful detention.

This true story of a German with a diploma, to whom I still have good contact to this day, was a prime example for me of the consequences that a poor medical history or a bad doctor-patient relationship can have.

I was inevitably reminded of this incident by a constructed example from the book of medical psychology by Prof. Dr. Goeppert:

A young man from a small, remote village in a developing country is uprooted from his familiar environment due to a political upheaval in his homeland and, as a result of various coincidental circumstances, is flown to a highly industrialized country. There, he, along with many others, leaves the airport and is hit by a car while crossing a busy street a few minutes later. He loses consciousness. When he comes to, he finds himself in a room with other people, all of whom have white skin. He is in great pain. In this new environment, he feels fear and wants to leave the room if possible. He struggles to get up. After succeeding, a woman dressed in white rushes toward him, speaks to him in an unfamiliar language, and tries to put him back to bed. When he desperately resists, she calls for someone, and a man dressed in white arrives to help her force him back into bed against his will. The young man realizes that it is not possible to flee at this moment. He waits in fear for what will happen next. Shortly thereafter, two women enter the room and distribute food to some of the people. The young man, like a few others, is given nothing. At first, he had no clear idea of his current, strange situation. After being forcibly prevented from leaving the room, he is convinced that he is in a hostile environment. This theoretical assumption is suggested by the unfamiliar surroundings and by the injury from the car accident. He has not seen anyone deliberately do anything bad to him yet. However, when he is not given food while others around him are, he perceives this as a deliberately hostile act. He notices that some of the white people in the room also do not receive food. He sees them as, at least in part, fellow sufferers, and watches their behavior with great interest. He observes that those who have not received food seem much more tense, anxious, and nervous than the people who have been given food. Along with his previous experiences, this strengthens his belief that he is facing an unpleasant fate, brought about by hostile people. Shortly thereafter, a man enters and pushes the bed of one of the white people who have not been given food out of the room. During this action, the great anxiety on the man's face is clearly visible. This event also reinforces the certainty that the people without food are being led to an unpleasant fate, and this observation fits well with the theoretical assumptions he has developed so far.

Soon after, the young man sees an empty bed being pushed past the window of the room. He suspects that this is the bed of the white man who was recently taken out. Later, when another man is taken out of the room, he already expects that an empty bed will soon be pushed past the window. In fact, his prediction, based on his theory, proves correct. An empty bed is pushed past, and with great horror, he sees a large bloodstain on one side of the bed. Now, it seems to him that the people who have not received food are being taken away and, as the blood suggests, killed. The empty beds are then transported elsewhere. Terrified, the young man tries to escape again, but this is prevented by a woman and a man who comes to her aid.

After lying frozen in terror for some time, hope begins to stir in him once more. Perhaps these were different beds being pushed past the window. He thinks about how he might verify this, wondering whether it is the beds of the people who were taken away that he sees rolled past the window shortly afterward. To confirm this, he tears a piece of his bed sheet and wraps it around the side of the bed of his neighbor, who also did not receive any food. After some time, this neighbor is taken away, and shortly afterward, he sees the bed with the white fabric strip wrapped around it, passing by the window. Now, he is certain that the people who have not received food are being taken somewhere else and killed. He will think further about why this might be happening. Based on his experience, he might think of human sacrifice, hatred of white people towards others, or even cannibalism. When his own bed is finally rolled out, he has resigned himself to death. He is taken to a small room, where there are again white-clad women and men. They turn to him and begin handling strange instruments. Finally, he smells a strange odor and begins to feel sleepy. His last thought is that his death does not seem to be painful.

This example illustrates the following: A person is generally unable to make observations without preconceived notions. They have certain expectations and want to integrate new observations into their existing worldview. The mental constructs, the theoretical ideas, do not arise directly from the data; rather, at least some of the ideas were already present beforehand.

When comparing the two examples, I considered the constructed example more likely, as I still find the first one hard to believe. On the other hand, this serves as an important lesson about how crucial a medical history is, even in a homogeneous culture, and the difficulties and misunderstandings that arise when attempting to adopt practices from other cultures.

I would like to remind that a hospital, with all its facilities, is still a foreign institution for the average African. The example of the "young man" from the small village applies similarly regardless of whether the hospital in Africa has African staff although not as acute. The question now is: what goes through the mind of an African when they are admitted to a hospital?

How should one best take a medical history from them or establish a good doctor-patient relationship? How should one approach them so that they do not flee the hospital but instead remain cooperative and take their medication?

Thus, we are already talking about patient compliance: a major issue not only in Africa but also in industrialized countries. Jansen writes:

"Compliance with medical treatment has been a topic for much discussion in world literature since the 195O's. 'The reliability of the patient in taking the therapy must be a fundamental consideration' (Bonnar & Goldberg, 1969). Gradually it has been accepted that a doctor treating a patient with certain drugs cannot take it for granted that his instructions and prescriptions are fully followed through. The majority of these compliance studies refer to western medical practices. It is discouraging to take stock of the compliance rate of treatment schedules under intra-cultural conditions. Davis (1968) reviewing 31 publications dealing with this problem of noncompliance, states that the percentage of patients failing to follow up their doctor's orders varied between 15-93%. A review of this literature may help us to understand the defaulting that occurs in self-administration of drugs. Charney et co-workers (1967) collected figures from seven pediatric private practices in Rochester, New York. Only 56% of the children completed the prescribed ten-days course of oral penicillin. The authors suggested at the end of their article: 'Finally the most impressive correlations seem related to aspects of the patient-doctor relationship".[ix]

In Africa, the problem of "compliance" holds a special significance, in addition to the shortage of doctors and medications. Compliance is a sine qua non for the success of various WHO programs and development aid, as well as local government measures, aimed at improving medical care. Jansen has attempted to analyze this problem using the example of tuberculosis (TB) patients.

"When we opened our Ncihana clinic in 1968, we met a few members of a S.A.N.T.A. committee who were willing to assist us with TB. Control work. In January 1969 we appointed three of them, one man and two middle-aged women as home visitors. They were literate people and lived in the vicinity of our Ncihana clinic. At the beginning of the following month, they reported their findings to us. In Table 5 the data collected from these home visits are diagrammatically represented.

This pattern of reasons and excuses reported to our home visitors reflect generally the daily affairs of Bantu life. It is an open question as to whether the reasons reported correspond with the real situation at home or were made-up answers to satisfy the home-visitor or doctor. What we experienced was that most patients gave similar reasons to us when they came again to our clinic, so most are likely to be true and therefore it is important to reflect upon them. Social affairs keep tribal people busy and cause a number of them to be away from home for a couple of weeks or more."[x]

Even more interesting is the comment made by Jansen:

"Sickness at home is always a highly emotional affair to the Bomvana and under such circumstances he feels obliged to stay with his sick people in the hut as evidence of strong participation".

Trivial reasons together with "no excuse" formed the greatest category of defaulters (27.8%). It may be that psychological barriers contributed on this undefined group. One patient who did not attend our TB. clinic for months told us that his donkey had run away and now he had made efforts to seek and fetch it. Others only confessed to us: Ndimathile (I'm stupid). Perhaps it can be translated into modern language as: "IT have no internal motivation to attend the clinic". Of course, the category of no excuse! is a heterogeneous group of people who do not wish to reveal their reasons for non-attendance or had unconscious resistance to the treatment. Summing up the results of this survey, we are confronted with a very complex problem because the whole of tribal life is involved in causing the irregularity in attendance for chemotherapy.

Roelsgaard et al. (1964) who made an epidemiological study of tuberculosis in Africa stated:

"How this psychological barrier in self-administration of drugs is to be overcome is perhaps the biggest single question that has to be answered in the control of tuberculosis in developing areas" (p. 476).

A more critical situation arose when the relatives of a patient came to fetch him (called *uku-boleka* = to borrow) or when the patient himself requested his discharge at a time when the doctor did not want to disrupt the hospital treatment. Several reasons motivated the relatives to fetch such a patient. The first group of reasons was associated with the fact that the relatives regarded the condition of the patient as unsatisfactory. The deterioration of his general state or a mental change were indications for them to look out for other means of treating him. "There is apparently something of isi-Xhosa involved in his illness", the people argued to us. "We are satisfied with your treatment", they said, "and you have done your best, but something else must be done at home".[xi]

Jansen is right when he claims that "the whole tribal life is involved in causing the irregularity for the chemotherapy." However, he has overlooked another fact: namely, the whole of tribal life is involved in causing THE REGULARITY in attendance of any therapy. This remark is important in that it has practical consequences, which to this day many doctors in Africa have not recognized. I will return to this important point later. Jansen is only partially right when he further explains that "the first reason why patients do not come for treatment, is tribal medicine."

He reflects the widespread belief that compliance is low because of the medicine men. Nevertheless, "tribal medicine" or the medicine man is a secondary reason for non-compliance. I believe that one must investigate the primary reason further in order to properly understand the issue.

John M. Janzen also questioned "tribal medicine" as a cause:

'Medical writers on African medical practices such as Gelfand, Harley, and most recently Jansen, have transported their Western conception of the physician normatively confronting an individual sufferer to African settings, where native therapy is reported as if the same thing occurs there. This perspective creates an illusion that traditional specialists have superficial functions within the society. It leads one of these writers, for example, to suggest that once witch doctors have been suppressed by 'civilization,' the deleterious fear of witchcraft will disappear. However, if, as we propose in this study, norms and beliefs concerning illness and therapy are profoundly coded into the lives and minds of sufferers and their kinsmen, friends, and neighbors, the theoretical and practical issues of medical usages come into quite another perspective. The therapy-managing group phenomenon becomes a generic concept with probably universal representation in all societies."

G. Jansen reports with concern:

'We remember vividly children with severe dehydration being on intravenous drips whose mothers came back the day after admission to fetch them. The old people or the father had blamed the mother for leaving her child at the hospital without consulting them."

As he correctly pointed out, "sickness at home is always a highly emotional affair," and as I said, compliance is also a "family affair." The right thing to do would be, for example, to admit the child to the hospital, but even during the anamnesis, one should find out who is in charge at home. After Jansen had learned this, he was able to tell the mother that the doctor urgently wanted to speak with the responsible person the next day. The doctor's contact with the "responsible" person would be seen as a sign of respect for authority, and if this were regularly practiced in this way, people would view the doctor as someone who respects their customs, and this would be the beginning of trust.

I hope it is becoming clearer when I suggest adapting procedures that are recognized in conventional medicine to African circumstances. I see no good prospects for the implementation of various WHO programs or any health programs if there is no strategy in place that ensures these measures align with village life.

I would like to highlight the difference between conventional medicine and African reality using a quote. Prof. Dr. Goeppert describes:

"In our present-day society, in which healthcare is situated in the tension between the rule-of-law principles, where the state fulfills more or less static guardian functions, and the welfare-state system thinking with a tendency towards planning and directing social behavior, the primary goal is to normatively regulate the disease behavior of the population in such a way that it is directed towards rapid recovery and reintegration into society. This is primarily done by defining illness as a deviation from the socially accepted norm and through the institutionalized complementarity of the formal roles of doctor and patient in the doctor-patient relationship, which Parsons (1951, Chapter 10) characterized through four features in terms of rights and duties:

1. The doctor explains to the patient that they are not responsible for their illness by diagnosing it as a medical condition that cannot be fully understood and overcome by the patient's individual capabilities alone.
2. Precisely because the patient, as a layperson, is not able to adequately assess their illness, they are obligated to seek competent help from the expert doctor and cooperate with them.
3. The doctor legitimizes the patient in temporarily not fulfilling their responsibilities in the family, work, and other roles.
4. The doctor's role exemption due to illness also includes the patient's obligation to recover as quickly as possible.

Specifically, the patient must, in any case, demonstrate the will to get well.

In this systems-theoretical and functionalist concept of the formal, strictly complementary roles of doctor and patient (doctor = expert and authority - patient = layperson and help-seeking sick individual), the illness is seen as a static condition, deviating from normative values of the patient.

The uniqueness of our worldview (and therefore a special anamnesis) and our family structure led to a different patient role compared to Western medicine. As African doctors, we are familiar with both systems, and we must recognize the difference. In our case, points 1 and 3 of the above quote do not apply, and point 4 only partially. This difference is not just academic.

If the doctor applied the above-mentioned doctor-patient role to an average African patient, this patient would feel the doctor's attitude. The patient would either not accept the treatment or, as is usually the case, try to reach a compromise. However, this would create a difficulty for "real information" or anamnesis. The following quote from Jansen actually illustrates the doctor-patient role where the patient made such a compromise:

"Another aspect of the communication problem is that when a Bomvana patient consults a European doctor, he has already unconsciously chosen the less mythical approach for the relief of his suffering. In other words, he has chosen the somatic escape as the most efficient solution of his problem. This hampers a comprehensive psychosomatic approach to these indigenous patients."[xxii]

In some parts of Africa, the patient's "patient role" is first determined by the family, and the family (point 3 from Goeppert) "legitimizes them to temporarily refrain from fulfilling their duties in family and work and other role obligations." I cannot emphasize this difference enough, as it is deeply rooted in our society. I believe that the determination of the patient role by the family brings many advantages, with the doctor providing support and serving as an advisor through their expertise. The doctor can accept this defined doctor-patient role without compromising their medical art, leaving enough room for active cooperation with the patient and their family to overcome the illness. This type of patient role is brilliantly presented by John M. Janzen in his chapter "The Clan as Patient."

Before I close this chapter, I would like to express my conviction that I have great hope for medicine in Africa. Let us not see mythology, witchcraft, etc., as the greatest barrier to Western medicine: they are not! Let us remember that Christianity came to us, and despite its great differences from our concepts of God or gods, many Africans are Christians today. "There is no second continent that is as strongly shaped by religion as Africa. Unlike in Europe, the figures provided are not a convention... about 38% are Christians, with 60 million people being counted... Nearly 20% belong to the group of so-called Animists, that is, to traditional African nature religions."

Here is evidence of the plasticity or the possibility of changing negative health concepts fostered by mythology. But unlike in the past with Christianity, we Africans no longer blindly give up everything, including the positive. It is said, "if one finger is dirty, you don't cut off the whole hand." We Africans are willing to sacrifice a lot for our health as we have always done with the medicine man but we insist that our needs, which do not contradict health, continue to be respected. Some of these needs were addressed by the medicine man,

This leads me to my next chapter. What exactly did the medicine man do? What can we as doctors learn from this without compromising our art?

Further Reading

1. A.B. Chilivumbo, ***Medical Anthropology, Social Basis of Illness: A Search for Therapeutic Meaning***, USA: Mouton Publishers, 1976, p. 75 ff
2. MJ. Field, ***Search for Security***, USA: Northwestern University Press, 1962, p. 13
3. Paul Parin, ***Der Widerspruch im Subjekt, Ethnopsychoanalytische Studien***, Frankfurt am Main, Syndikat, 1978, p. 150
4. Albert Schweitzer, ***Selbstzeugnisse***, Munich: Verlag C.H. Beck, 1967, p. 193
5. G. Jansen, ***The Doctor-Patient-Relationship in an African Tribal Society***, Assen: Van Gorcum & Comp. B.V, 1973, p. 76
6. Cf. MJ. Field, ***Search for Security***, as cited, p. 144
7. Paul Hinderling, ***Ist der Medizinmann ein Devinator, Exorzist, ...? In: Curare, Zeitschrift für Ethnomedizin und transkulturelle Psychiatrie***, Vol. 4, 1981, p. 123

8. Jurgen Dahmer, ***Anamnese und Befund. Die systematische ärztliche Untersuchung***, Stuttgart: Georg Thieme Verlag, 1981, p. 13
9. Sebastian Goeppert, ***Medizinische Psychologie***, Vol. 1, Rowohlt Taschenbuch Verlag GmbH, 1980, p. 22-23
10. John M. Janzen, ***The Quest of Therapy in Lower Zaire***, USA: University of California Press, 1978, p. 7
11. Cf. G. Jansen, ***The Doctor-Patient-Relationship in an African Tribal Society***, as cited, p. 158
12. S. Goeppert, ***Medizinische Psychologie***, Vol. 2, Rowohlt Taschenbuch Verlag GmbH, 1980, p. 184-185
13. Cf. John M. Janzen, ***The Quest of Therapy in Lower Zaire***, as cited, p. 114 ff
14. Cf. Christoph von Imhoff, ***Jesus ist der Befreier, Muntu und der Gott der Christen sind eins - Die unabhangigen afrikanischen Kirchen ein Politikum, In: Das Parlament***, January 13, 1979, p. 20

Notes

[ix] Cf. G. Jansen, ***The Doctor-Patient-Relationship in an African Tribal Society***, as cited, p. 147-148

[x] Cf. G. Jansen, ***The Doctor-Patient-Relationship in an African Tribal Society***, as cited, p. 154-155

[xi] Cf. G. Jansen, ***The Doctor-Patient-Relationship in an African Tribal Society***, as cited, p. 156-157

[xii] Cf. G. Jansen, ***The Doctor-Patient-Relationship in an African Tribal Society***, as cited, p. 82

CHAPTER II

WHO IS THE MEDICINE MAN?

1. Objections and Considerations about Medicine Men and Doctors (Traditional Medicine)

What has he really done, or what does he do? But before I write about the medicine man, I would like to address some objections that exist against this topic. Therefore, the reader must excuse me for making a digression here first. *The Journal of General Medicine* (ZFA) dedicated an entire issue to the topic "The Science of Non-Science." For example, Wolf Wimmer, in the article "Witchcraft Delusion at Universities?", claims that Prof. Dr. Hans Bender, former chair of "Border Areas of Psychology," and his successor Prof. Dr. John Mischo had dedicated themselves to "ghost research."

"The science of ghosts actually exists. It is called parapsychology and can be studied at the University of Freiburg in Breisgau."

"In other words: empirically confirmed facts, which are long-established knowledge of the natural sciences, no longer require proof. Rather, the burden of proof lies with those who wish to dispute them. I do not have to repeatedly prove, for example, that the Earth is a sphere and that an apple falls from a tree. This seems entirely self-evident to any sane person. However, occultists think differently."

Although the objections here are directed against parapsychology, similar arguments are often heard at conferences or among colleagues when discussing the topic of the "medicine man."

Unfortunately, the arguments made by Wolf Wimmer seem weak to me. One only needs to point out that many axioms of Newtonian physics and Euclidean geometry were accepted as self-evident for a very long time. In these two scientific fields, the evidence (if I may use the term) is even "more evident" than the evidence in psychology. Nevertheless, those "earlier evidences" were supplemented or corrected by theories such as relativity and quantum mechanics. No serious scientist can categorically deny that there will still be revolutions in the so-called natural sciences in the future, whereby today's accepted truths may be questioned or changed. Why shouldn't this also apply to psychology or medicine?

I would also like to point out that similar questions, as those posed about the "Freiburg ghost research," have also been raised and continue to be raised in the United States. For example, the "International Foundation for Biosocial Development and Human Health" states:

"There appears to be a growing sentiment that the practice of medicine has reached some sort of dangerous fork in the road."

The two major complaints appear to revolve around the accelerating high cost of the delivery of medical services and an increasing depersonalization of the doctor-patient-relationship. Further reflection on both of these criticisms suggest that the problems are to some extent associated with the tremendous advances in technology over the past two decades. The metastasizing spread of the computer into all phases of medical diagnosis and treatment, development of sophisticated hardware and instrumentation appear to have made medicine more and more of a science and less a personalized art that addresses the patient as in individual.

In reaction or rebellion to this trend, and spurred on by an increasing wariness and fear of the unknown term and side effects of medication as well as ecological hazards associated with scientific advances, patients in droves are turning towards naturopathic or holistic modalities of therapy, particularly if they can be demonstrated to be physiologic or non-toxic.

Surely there must be some solution to this. There must be some method via which physicians and patients can enjoy the fruits of scientific research but still retain that personalized partnership which is the magic and mystery of the healing art of medicine.

There are all sorts of information floating around out there, information accumulating at an hourly rate. Information about scientific and technology advances about verifiable parapsychological phenomena such as faith healing, about how the body can utilize its innate potential to heal itself and how the physician can synergize that process, about the powers of the mid and the role of the brain as an awesome endocrine organ as well as a complex electronic network. To be utilized meaningfully it must be communicated to the scientific community as soon as possible so that it can be evaluated and integrated and incorporated in a larger body of meaningful knowledge and again communicated to the appropriate recipient.

In the final analysis, good health is simply a matter of effective communication internally between the constituent components of the organism in its efforts to maintain the constancy and integrity of the internal environment in response to stress, and meaningful communication between the individual and the external environment. If you think about it, the same may be said for a single cell, a nation of a society, as well as a profession such as medicine."[xiii]

When I read arguments against "pseudo-science, medicine men, and witchcraft," I am spontaneously reminded of my school days, where our teacher, in an introduction to philosophy, told us: "*Si philosophandum est, philosophandum est, etiam si non philosophandum est, philosophandum est, utinam,*" etc. At the time, this was a critique of the Sophists, who rejected philosophy *a priori.*

The point was that if it is necessary to philosophize, then one must philosophize, and even if it is not necessary to philosophize, one must philosophize to demonstrate that philosophizing is not necessary. In other words, philosophizing must always be done. Similarly, it should be permissible to discuss pseudo-science, witchcraft, medicine men, and so on. One only needs to attempt to view the topic without bias to open the possibility for new approaches.

Another important reason for me to speak about the "medicine man" is that it is a current topic, and one should not simply turn a blind eye to this fact: it is a reality that the medicine man is still present in Africa.

"We have other examples of the ways officials consult banganga, give them patronage, and use them as agents of social control. Political figures, of whatever level in government, feel pressures and hostilities against them, and seek protection or clarification of their situation from ritual experts. The cases out here suggest that ritual power is an important option used by officials. They tell us something about the nganga's role and the confidence political figures have in ritual power. When a particular nganga has established himself as a charismatic authority, he becomes an available tool and vehicle of governmental process. The legitimation is personalized in that an individual nganga gives ritual support to a political figure who then gives him protection. A Kongo proverb describes the relationship" "Chiefs are chiefs; magicians are Magicians" (mfumu na mfumu, nganga na nganga), meaning that they work together, each in his own way. In the words of the commissioner of national security in Thysville on the pass permit, "I request all military and civilian authorities to aid and abet him in every need."[xiv]

Or, as J. Neumann puts it: "Anyone working in the medical field in Africa faces the confrontation between indigenous healing practices and European culture." It is also a fact that the UN's World Health Organization (WHO) repeatedly recommends integrating traditional medicine and indigenous doctors (medicine men) into the healthcare systems of the respective developing countries. For example, in the "*Serie de Rapport Techniques de I'Organisation Mondiale de la Sante, " Bureau Regional de I'Afrique, No. 1, 1976*, the following can be read:

"The necessity and opportunity of integrating the activities of traditional healers into those of health services, particularly concerning primary healthcare.

Status of Traditional Medicine

According to information received from 19 countries in the African Region:

- **8 countries** have, at the level of the Ministry of Health, a unit dedicated to traditional medicine.
- **13 countries** carry out significant activities in the field of traditional medicine, either in the form of applied research, treatments prescribed by physicians in conjunction with traditional medicine, or through the involvement of traditional healers within the traditional framework, whether integrated into the health team or collaborating more or less closely with it.
- **10 countries** have institutes, research centers, and herbaria focused on issues related to traditional medicine.
- **6 countries** conduct research in this field within universities.
- **5 countries** have designated national commissions responsible for traditional medicine issues or have organized

national colloquiums, conferences, workshops, and seminars on the subject.

- **7 countries** have officially recognized traditional medicine associations.
- **3 countries** have legislation on traditional medicine.

Possibilities for Integration

Having recognized the impact of traditional medicine on health in Africa, the Committee acknowledged the necessity and opportunity of integrating its activities into various health services. However, given the historical conditions prevailing thus far between the two medical systems, their differing fundamental concepts, and their methods, which are not easily aligned, such an integration of their activities can only be envisioned and implemented very gradually, with the utmost attention paid to the specific conditions of each region or country.[xv]

A year later, this recommendation for "traditional medicine" was brought back into discussion:

"The purpose of the meeting was therefore to bring together specialists from the main traditional medical systems and have them work together on developing an action plan for the promotion and development of the various elements that make up this form of medicine."[xvi]

As in almost all African countries, medicine men flourished everywhere, including in Mozambique, despite legal prohibitions. The population would not dare to denounce a medicine man to the authorities. Last but not least, a phenomenon observed across Africa was that even the colonialists eventually sought out the medicine men.

The inconsistencies of the colonial state naturally did not contribute to driving the medicine men away.

"The colonial authorities were inconsistent; healers were harassed by some officials for a period and yet permitted to practice at other times. Colonial officials even protected the work of the banganga. On rare occasions, and in a few instances, Europeans are said to have consulted the banganga in a clandestine manner. The prevailing view of the officials was that banganga were no great harm, and perhaps even useful in maintaining order. When Catholic and Protestant missionaries complained, however, they would investigate and harass or imprison individual practitioners. This approach to the banganga contrasted to the treatment of bangunza, whom Belgian colonialists sought out with a paranoia unequalled in other colonial systems. Virtually all individuals who drew attention as ngunza were imprisoned, exiled, or kept under surveillance until 1958. The Belgians feared massive insubordination and saw these religious leaders as a real political threat. In 1921, Kimbangu, the most celebrated prophet, was sentenced to death and then imprisoned for life in Katanga, where he died in 1951. Other prophets were exiled to work camps in the Upper Congo."[xvii]

Over time, the population noticed the differing success of treatments from traditional and Western medicine. As a result, some African patients had certain ideas about the different types of doctors, as J. Neumann also observed.

Hospital Doctor	**Native Doctor**	**Wizard**
Pulmonary disease Sterility Psychiatric illness Sexually transmitted diseases (STDs) Diseases that require surgery Wounds Eye diseases Ear pain	Sterility Epilepsy Jaundice Liver disease Toothache	Pulmonary disease Psychiatric illness Diseases caused by conflicts with other people Physical weakness

This classification is, of course, not representative of all of Africa, but the idea that one group of diseases can only be cured by traditional medicine, a second group of diseases can only be cured by modern medicine, and a third group of diseases cannot be attributed to either traditional or modern medicine.

"In some countries, indeed, diseases have been classified into three broad categories - those curable by indigenous medicine, those curable by modern medicine, and those that are self-limiting, and not affected by either indigenous or modern medicine."

The existence of both traditional medicine and modern medicine forces me to ask whether the two systems could collaborate. In addition to the already mentioned WHO recommendations for cooperation between traditional and modern medicine, one can read the following for example:

"The meeting of indigenous peoples with the science of ancient cultures, and even with the knowledge of Europe since the Age of Discovery, has not fundamentally changed their therapeutic methods, but it has changed some aspects. For example, Malaysian medicine men, as recent studies by Wolfgang Week on Bali have shown, have been significantly influenced by India and China, and are not entirely closed off to European medicine. It is even possible for cooperation with European doctors, who have acquired the necessary knowledge of language, country, and people, and earned the necessary trust. Joint efforts to combat epidemics, with an understanding of modern hygiene, have also been observed (Seiffert)."

Or an example from China:

"There is no clear gradation from one level of health worker to another in China.

Nonetheless it is possible to divide China's health workers into rough categories:

Full-time workers:

- Higher medical Workers:
  - Doctors of Western medicine.
  - Stomatologists
  - Pharmacologists
  - Doctors of Chinese medicine

Middle medical workers:

- Assistant doctors
- Nurses
- Midwives
- Pharmacists
- Technicians

Part-time workers:

- Barefoot doctors
- Worker doctors
- Red medical workers

Spare-time workers:

- Health aides"

The education of doctors of Western medicine has undergone profound changes in recent years. Since the Cultural Revolution, considerable emphasis has been placed in all medical schools on teaching traditional medicine. In some cities, such as Nanking, the former traditional medical college has been combined with a Western type medical college; in others, such as Kwangchow and Peking, the two types of college have informal links, and some graduates of Western medical colleges may attend traditional colleges for further work after graduation.

Perhaps the most difficult assessment in this analysis is the degree to which China's experience is applicable to other developing countries. It is often said that because of China's social, economic, political and cultural circumstances differ so markedly from those of other countries, there is little in the Chinese experience that can be directly transferred. While this may be true and Chinese representatives have themselves frequently stated that each country must find solutions to its problems based on its own special circumstances there are basic principles that may indeed be relevant to other societies. These include the emphasis on local self-reliance, on brief training and structured part-time use of locally recruited and locally trained people, on the combination of modern and traditional medicine, and on preventive medicine. Perhaps even more important if difficult to implement are the beliefs that fundamental changes in health and health care may require fundamental changes in the social structure in which they are embedded, that equitable distribution of resources must be a basic goal of society, and that the opportunity to be of service should be a prime motivating force in health work as in other human services. But surely the greatest lesson that China offers is that it can be dome - that a nation can within one generation move from a starving, sickness-riddled, illiterate, Elitist semi-feudal society to a vigorous, healthy, productive, highly literate, mass participation society. If China can accomplish it, other nations can too."[xviii]

We do not need to imitate everything from China or other health systems, but we can benefit from some of their successes. In my opinion, for cooperation with traditional medicine, a realistic analysis of what one wants to achieve and how a program should be developed to implement it is necessary. However, this requires personal commitment to both traditional and Western medicine; competence and 'diplomacy' are essential to integrate the positive aspects of both systems into a program and meet the needs of the population. As long as all of this is lacking, as is often the case with such projects today, the warning from Prof. Dr. Diesfeld is likely to be appropriate:

"Since five years and increasingly since the Alma-Ata Conference on Primary Health Care in 1978, the World Health Organization has been programmatically calling for 'Health (Primary Health Care)' for all by the year 2000.' However, it is clear to all experts in the field, and likely to the political authorities as well, that this will hardly be achievable in the available 20 years, especially if the political conditions are not created at the national level.

Primarily brought into the public spotlight through the example of China, traditional medicine has also gained more significance in international circles. Thus, in the call for primary health care for all by the year 2000, traditional medicine has been included in the calculation. This represents an acknowledgment of the modern medicine's inability to meet the health care demands. However, it simultaneously constitutes a hollow political formula in global health policy, because from this perspective, 'Primary Health Care for all' has always existed. If the year 2000 is set as a target, one can only hope that, in the course of its official recognition and the intended 'integration,' traditional medicine will not be legally formalized to death by then."

Danger for Traditional Medicine?

One can only hope that 20 years of administration and bureaucracy will not achieve what 200 years of colonialism did not accomplish. There is a fear that the administrative consequences of the health policy demand for decentralization of modern health care and the integration of traditional medicine, along with the subtle forms of scientific cultural and social anthropology, ethnology, and ethnomedicine field research, combined with the general cultural upheaval, will completely and permanently destroy traditional medicine.

Health Care Only for the Elites

Why should this happen, when the advocates for a return to cultural values see it as an opportunity to rediscover cultural identity? Until now, there have been two largely separate worlds in a pronounced medical pluralism, where the patient had to choose among them. There has always been, and so far rarely broken, a multifaceted system of traditional medicine, which since the colonial era was initially fought against by Western medicine and Christian churches, and later disregarded. It then became clear that the majority of the population was medically meaning, Western medically undersupplied.

Modern Medicine Remained a Foreign Body

Every culture and civilization have its concept of health, illness, and healing according to its knowledge and understanding, and thus a corresponding health or medical care system. Like so much else, the countries of the former colonies were presented with a foreign medical system along with all its advantages and disadvantages through foreign penetration. However, it has remained largely a foreign body to this day, except for the few who participated in the colonial and post-colonial acculturation and development process.

On the other hand, traditional healers pragmatically use the symbols of modern medicine, such as stethoscopes and syringes, and also use modern medications. With the blending of systems, the door has understandably been opened to fraud, charlatanism, and quackery, to the detriment of both systems and especially the patients.

Here lies a great danger. The well-meaning attempt to bring the systems closer together can lead to the weaker system being overwhelmed by the stronger one, completely altered, and ultimately eradicated, without equivalent replacement being provided.

Here, a good deed can become a curse. Therefore, a rational discussion between both systems must be conducted with the necessary moral seriousness and mutual respect. Whether the first international conference on traditional medicine in Canberra in 1979 and the international association of traditional healers will mark a positive turning point remains to be seen. However, this area must certainly be taken into account within the framework of health aid by the federal government and non-governmental health aid organizations, which, however, requires stronger advocacy from the working groups dealing with issues of intercultural comparative health research, ethnomedicine, and medical anthropology.

Thus, the reader should be aware of the relevance of this topic, although I would like to mention that I have excluded the studies of some scientists on the treatment success of traditional healers in schizophrenic patients to avoid deviating too far from the focus of this work.

2. The Complexity of the Term "Medicine Man" and His Services

I believe that both the above quotes and the efforts in Africa regarding traditional medicine raise the question: Who is the medicine man?

This is a question that provides enough material to write an entire book. Dr. Paul Hinderling from the Social Psychological Unit for Development Planning at the University of Saarland wrote the following about the complexity of this topic: "Is the medicine man a diviner, exorcist, healer, witch doctor, herbalist, cult leader, oracle, shaman, seer, fortune teller, or magician?" Each of these designations is somewhat applicable, but certain limitations must be made, depending on which continent, country, and tribe the medicine man is from.

Therefore, I will only address the most important aspects of the term "medicine man" as they are relevant to this work.

The medicine man is primarily a healer, and it is believed that he manipulates "with some magical powers, most of all with magical (partly symbolic, partly medically efficient) means of assistance." The medicine man is a fighter against illness, and for us Africans, he is the one who knows the secrets of healing and, therefore, inevitably the secrets of "causing sickness."

Therefore, it is believed that the medicine man can cause diseases with "symbolic and magical powers." The latter characteristic of the medicine man is secondary. However, for foreign researchers, especially for the colonizers of Africa, these two abilities were so striking that they placed primary emphasis on the ability to "cause illness." As a result, the medicine man was unfairly referred to as a "Witchdoctor" in English and as "Cuchucnucheiro" (slang) or "feticetro" in Portuguese. Today, young intellectual Africans still try to present the medicine man primarily as a healer.

"... Although everyone under cover of darkness treks to them (traditional healers), our men of medicine who have brought us thus far are still to us only witch doctors, the same way as colonialists."

In my tribe (as in many other African tribes), the terms medicine man' and 'witch doctor' are clearly distinguished. The medicine man, diviner, magician, "witch doctor" is depicted as follows:

Medicine Man	Diviner
Healer	Priest-doctor
Diviner	Healer
Wizard	Wizard

Wizard	Witchdoctor
Witchdoctor	Wizard
Healer	Diviner
Diviner	Healer

In my tribe, as well as in many other patriarchal tribes, one becomes a medicine man through "inheritance," and the training period begins early in childhood. Similar customs can be found in Madagascar, which lies opposite Mozambique.

"The medicine men acquire their knowledge over a long training period of 5 to 15 years under elder masters."

When a patient visited the medicine man, the entire family was usually present and actively participated in the treatment. For example, dancing and communal singing are integral parts of the healing process:

"Music is extraordinarily widespread in the treatment of the sick."

Or as Jansen observes:

"We remember a little boy of four years old who once entered our clinic with his mother and asked in amazement: 'When is this doctor going to start dancing?' For dancing (*uku-xhensa*) is the main activity of the diviner during the séance."

After the dance, the medicine man often places his hands on the patient, while the relatives wait anxiously for the diagnosis and prognosis. Frequently, the "diagnosis" is simultaneously the "etiology" and vice versa. Here, the role as a diviner takes precedence, and the cause of the illness in some cases is attributed to the dissatisfaction of a deceased family member or a spirit or deity.

Often, a sacrifice, such as a chicken on the grave, suffices.

"The belief that illness arises from supernatural causes and indicates the displeasure of ancestral gods and evil spirits or is the effect of black magic is still held by many communities in developing countries. To deal with such causes, indigenous healers undertake elaborate exorcising rituals on behalf of the sick and mentally affected."

As the quote suggests, "black magic" or "witchcraft" is often diagnosed as the cause of illness, with a relative of the patient frequently being blamed. This is an aggressive diagnosis, and the medicine man often risks his reputation and career in the process. The patient and their relatives expect the medicine man to simultaneously "guess" or explain how the conflict began, how it developed, and how it can be resolved.

Remarkably, misdiagnoses are rare, which is due to the highly developed anamnesis (medical history) process of the medicine man, as I will demonstrate later (see Chapter IV).

Ethnomedical literature recognizes the psychological impact of the medicine man; however, I believe this "mere recognition" is insufficient. It is even more important to investigate how the medicine man systematically gathers medical history and simultaneously uses it as a form of talk therapy. This type of anamnesis essentially a "talk therapy" is acceptable to the average African and provides a real chance for a strong doctor-patient relationship.

I would like to briefly say a few words about the achievements of the medicine men regarding their treatment of organic diseases. I will not categorize these achievements by tribe, as is done by various researchers, since no clear distinction is possible. For example, the medicine men of the Maasai tribe were admired as great surgeons, but there were also skilled surgeons in other tribes.

"The only tribe known to sure vessels (with tendons) is the Masai. We will encounter the Masai again and again as the primitive master of surgeons. They are atypical as their surgery is incomparable superior not only to that of other primitive tribes reported, but also to the surgery of most civilized peoples up to Renaissance.

The East African focus of good surgery is not limited to the Masai. Among their neighbors we have found such outstanding accomplishments as Caesarian section intestinal suture trepanation, excision of glands, etc."[xix]

Sometimes, after an operation in a Western hospital, the medicine man was consulted, especially when the patient's relatives were not satisfied with the results of the doctors. However, the success of the medicine man, particularly during the colonial period, was opposed by all means, as he was seen as competition and a threat to the system.

"The colonial reaction to indigenous therapy was sometimes very direct. As late as 1956, village healers in the Kibunzi and Mbanza Mwembe region were rounded up and reprimanded by colonial authorities after a patient had been removed by relatives from a mission hospital and taken to one of them. On the other occasion, a village herbalist was threatened with imprisonment and exile for removing the head of fetus from a woman who had attended a mission maternity ward where only the body had been born in a breach delivery."[xx]

Despite difficulties with the government and the church, the medicine men continued their work. The following is a somewhat incomplete table, but it still provides the reader with a small overview of the surgical services provided by the medicine men:

Ethnie bzw. Gebiet	**Operationstechnik / Art der Operation**	**Quellennachweis**
Massai	Wundnacht u. Gefäßnaht	Ackerknecht (1971), 96
"Nachbarn der Massai"	Darmnaht	l.c. 109
Uganda	Wundnaht	Bartels (1893), 283
Akamba	Wundnaht	Ackerknecht (1971), 96
Massai	Skarifikation, Einschnitte in die Tonsillen bei Mandelentzündung	l.c. 101
Massai	Enukleation des Auges bei schweren Augenverletzungen	l.c. 101
Massai	Entfernung von Abszessen aus Leber und Milz	l.c. 101
Massai	Amputation gebrochener Extremitäten; Prothesenanfertigung	l.c. 101
"Nachharn der Massai"	Kaiserschnitt Trepanation	l.c. 109
Uganda	Kaiserschnitt	l.c. 103 f. Bartels (1893), 305 f. Brandt (1966), 82 ff.
Uganda (auch in Nigeria)	Trepanation	Ackerknecht (1971), 104
Uganda	Amputation gebrochener Glieder	l.c. 108
Uganda	Anlegen eines Pneumothorax durch Brennen mit dem Brenneisen	l.c. 101
Barundi und Akamba	Öffnen von Abszessen mit dem Messer	l.c. 101

Ostafrika	Embryotomie (operative Zerstückelung des Kindes in der Gebärmutter bei Kindstod im Mutterleib oder bei absoluten Geburtshindernissen)	l.c. 104

Table adapted from Josef Neumann, 1978.

"This overview of the surgical techniques and healing methods commonly practiced in East Africa demonstrates that the African ethnic groups living around Lake Victoria possess a highly developed surgical tradition, which they routinely use as a healing method. They are capable of successfully performing complex operations (such as cesarean sections, amputations, and trepanations) and employ advanced surgical techniques (wound suturing, intestinal suturing, and vascular suturing).

It is therefore not surprising that a report from Uganda describes a plastic surgery procedure in which a man who had sustained an abdominal wound from a spear was treated by inserting a curved, round-cut piece of gourd to support his internal organs."[xxi]

In his article about indigenous peoples, Ulf Lind reports on other achievements of the medicine men:

"It is remarkable that they practice active immunization against venomous snake bites by allowing themselves to be bitten by a less venomous snake.

The Maasai of East Africa also knew of an active vaccination method for cattle against lung disease."[xxii]

Some of the indispensable medications found in all Western clinics were also used by the medicine men:

"Strophanthin was discovered in the arrow poison of indigenous peoples, brought back from Africa by Livingstone, as was physostigmine, also known as eserine, a component of the Calabar bean."[xxiii]

"Diuretics, electrolytes, minerals, etc., were pragmatically used by some medicine men."[xxiv]

When comparing the medications or active substances used by the medicine man with those of conventional medicine, many similarities can be found, without calling into question the superiority of Western pharmacology.

Recently, I was deeply moved when Prof. Dr. Reisert, chief physician and director of the Medical Clinic at St. Vincentius Hospital, explained to us during our practical year how shock treatment has evolved. "In my time," the dynamic professor recounted, "when I was a student like you, it was said that adrenaline must always be administered in cases of shock. Today, we must first differentiate between the various types of shock, as in some cases, adrenaline is strictly contraindicated."

For example:

"Acute Vascular Circulatory Insufficiency (Shock, Collapse)

The term acute vascular circulatory insufficiency refers to a circulatory disturbance in individual organs or the entire organism due to an absolute or relative mismatch between the capacity of the arterial and/or venous vascular system and its filling.

From a hemodynamic standpoint, shock and collapse must be distinguished from one another, particularly as this distinction also has therapeutic implications.

In shock, there is poor peripheral circulation due to a high peripheral resistance caused by general vasoconstriction, whereas in collapse, peripheral resistance is reduced due to a weakening of vasomotor tone, and vascular dilation is generally present.

Based on these differences in the functional state of the blood vessels, Duesberg and Schroeder differentiate between **tension collapse** (with vasoconstrictive narrowing of large parts of the peripheral vascular system, excessive tension in the Windkessel region of the aorta or large vessels, and centralization of circulation' by limiting blood flow primarily to the heart and large vessels) and **relaxation** collapse, characterized by dilation in the capillary area."

The clinical signs of circulatory insufficiency, despite the pathogenic differences, are quite uniform:

In a state of shock, the skin and mucous membranes appear pale due to constriction of their blood vessels. The extremities feel cold and are livid-cyanotic, particularly in the peripheral areas. The patient has a tense, anxious, and restless expression, unless unconsciousness is present. In cases of severe dehydration, cramps may occur. The pulse, if palpable, is somewhat tense. The heart rate is increased. Systolic blood pressure is significantly lowered, diastolic pressure is normal or elevated, and the pulse amplitude is reduced. Breathing is accelerated.

Further clinical examination often reveals very faint heart sounds. In peripheral circulatory insufficiency, the veins are collapsed, whereas in cardiac-related circulatory insufficiency, they are often engorged.

Collapse shows several differences compared to the symptoms of shock (though, as mentioned earlier, it cannot always be distinctly separated from shock): The skin is covered with cold sweat, the formulas, which lasts for hours and hours, becomes obsessive. One must think that all of this has repercussions on the nervous system of individuals, especially those who are ill. To MELOTHERAPY, as therapy of rhythm, we must add CHOREOTHERAPY. In this, purely symbolic acts directed against evil spirits, which provoke illnesses, are accompanied by physical-psychic reactions caused by the stage performance, by heavy sweating, which detoxifies the body, and by the increase in adrenaline which, in turn, carries fatty acids and harmful waste products in the blood that are subsequently eliminated. But beyond a certain limit, the hormonal surge can provoke a kind of collective exaltation with manifestations of aggression, and thus one can explain that primitive peoples resorted to dance before going into war or hunting. CHOREOTHERAPY is at the heart of healing rituals."

In this chapter, I have not attempted to list everything the medicine man did. I only want to schematically provide a small amount of information about what he is, what he did, and what discussions or opinions exist in this context. Above all, I want to give colleagues an insight who might be confronted with traditional medicine in Africa and who had previously judged it *a priori* as "hocus-pocus."

3. Nihil Nocere

The highest principle in the doctor-patient relationship since Hippocrates is: "do everything for the patient's benefit, or, as a minimal requirement, neither harm the patient through action nor inaction." This medical professional ethic should never be forgotten, even in Africa.

Before I conclude this chapter, "Who is the Medicine Man," I want to emphasize that, even if one remains convinced that medicine men should disappear, medical implications that were or are historically connected to them must still be considered.

The following examples serve to illustrate these concluding remarks.

In my tribe, the use of spider webs during childbirth is a known practice. After my training, I considered this custom unhygienic and advised my patients to refrain from it. Indeed, some doctors discovered the same custom in Mexico and deemed it dangerous for both mother and child due to the risk of infection. The inhabitants of this Mexican village followed the doctors' recommendations, and consequently, this custom disappeared.

When the doctors finished their development service, the village was left without medical care. Later, it was observed that during the period when the village was without a doctor, infant mortality increased significantly. An investigation revealed that spider webs had antibiotic properties, which protected both the mother and child during childbirth:

"For example, in Mexico, traditional midwives have always covered the umbilical cord of newborns with spider webs. Western doctors judged this practice as dirty and dangerous until it was discovered that spider saliva and the webs themselves have antibiotic properties a fact long understood by traditional midwives."

Or another example: In many parts of Africa, women are considered "unclean" during menstruation. One day, a colleague asked me about the reason for this. I replied: "The explanation can vary from tribe to tribe. But when I think back to our gynecology lecture, I don't find this custom so unreasonable. Menstrual blood is a breeding ground for many bacteria, such as Koch's bacteria, gonococci, etc. In a society where hygienic conditions are still inadequate and antibiotics are unavailable, I find this custom functionally very significant."

In a textbook on gynecology, one reads:

"Even better results have been achieved with the bacteriological examination of menstrual blood. For this purpose, an occlusive pessary is inserted at the beginning of the period. The pessary remains in place for several hours. The blood collected in the pessary is used to prepare a bacterial culture (duration 2-4 weeks) and for animal testing for tuberculosis (duration 3-5 weeks). Good results require the special processing of the examination material by a bacteriologist. A single negative result from a menstrual blood sample does not definitively rule out genital tuberculosis. Therefore, repeated bacteriological examinations are necessary. If three results are negative, the likelihood of open genital tuberculosis is low. Bacteriological examinations (culture and animal testing) can also be performed on curettage material. In any case, a tuberculosis-positive bacteriological finding proves active and open genital tuberculosis.

The indication for menstrual blood examination exists when there is clinical suspicion of genital tuberculosis and is especially warranted if there is a history of tuberculosis exposure. Moreover, menstrual blood examination is indicated as a routine screening method for various active organ tuberculosis cases. For example, it has been possible to detect often undiagnosed active genital tuberculosis in cases of lung tuberculosis, peritoneal and mesenteric lymph node tuberculosis, uro-tuberculosis, skeletal and joint tuberculosis with varying frequency.

It should also be mentioned that the findings on menstrual excretion of tuberculosis bacteria and the associated risk of infection for others call for epidemic hygiene precautions.

Menstrual pads and tampons must be burned. Work in kitchens, restaurants, food production, etc., must be prohibited. These precautions are so important because in many cases, tuberculosis bacteria are shed with menstrual blood for years, even though the patient does not feel ill and is therefore not considered unfit for work."

If, in this context, menstruating women are regarded as "unclean," and one considers the hygienic conditions and morbidity rates in some regions of Africa, one can see how appropriate this practice is. This has nothing to do with the personality or dignity of women in our society.

There are many such traditional customs that, at first glance, seem nonsensical. However, upon further reflection, one often finds similar underlying reasons that are confirmed by modern medicine.

"For example, if a butcher who cuts his finger presses the adrenal gland of the slaughtered animal onto the wound to stop the bleeding, this becomes a perfectly rational action in light of pharmacological knowledge about the blood-clotting and vessel-constricting effects of adrenaline."

For a butcher in industrialized countries, this therapy may be entirely obsolete. However, if an average African farmer treats the same injury with the bleeding adrenal gland of an animal, it might be his only option. If there is a doctor in the village, he might be able to obtain a hemostatic medication; but the next time, the doctor might be absent, leaving the farmer completely helpless because he was discouraged from using his traditional "unhygienic" treatment method.

This is confirmed by the following:

"The tenacity with which the human heart clings to tradition is hardly more evident than at the sickbed. This explains why remnants of the oldest days of humanity whether instinctive and unconscious, consciously empirical, magical-animistic, or theurgical healing practices have survived in the nameless folk medicine of all times and peoples to this day.

They have endured the transformations that folk medicine, like scientific medicine, has undergone due to the influences of human environments, the constant shifts in the spirit of the times, nature and culture, religion and politics, the humanities and natural sciences, and the achievements of technology.

It is striking how many similarities and parallels exist in the folk medicine concepts and practices across various parts of the world. Some can be explained by the "elementary thoughts" that the German physician and ethnologist Adolf Bastian (1826—1905) referred to ideas common to all peoples, arising from the same human organization, about God, the soul, world order, and so on. Others must be attributed to borrowing and tradition in the dynamic history of humanity."

I believe it is important and beneficial to support traditional practices that have proven effective as treatment methods. This approach aligns with the worldview of the patient and helps to build trust.

Prof. Dr. Antonio Scarpa says:

"It is evident, for example, that the pharmacological powers of penicillin are not diminished if the administration of penicillin is accompanied by harmless prayers, propitiatory offerings, phenomena of magical transfer of illness, or the sacrifice of animals. In this way, an advantage is gained, as the pharmacological action is strengthened by the psychic effect of beneficial emotional shocks, resulting in psychosomatic reactions as a consequence."

Put differently: If I need to treat a patient with penicillin and they also suffer from restlessness, anxiety, boredom, or discontent, and I could alleviate these symptoms additionally with music, it would be better than treating the same patient with penicillin (depending on the clinic or treating physician) combined with tranquilizers or medications like Tramal, Atosil, Haldol, Noctamid, or Valium. I am certain that the reader would also choose the first treatment option, especially considering the side effects.

I once visited a psychiatric ward where patients were lying around almost everywhere, some partially naked and so drugged by medications that they appeared like drunkards. I told my colleague that psychotropic drugs are undoubtedly of great help in therapy, but without proper indication, they can become the pornography of medicine.

I clearly remember my surprise when I heard the following during a lecture:

"In the Federal Republic of Germany (FRG), approximately 15 percent of adults suffer from anxiety. Tranquilizers have almost become a staple food. With prolonged use, tranquilizers may possibly affect personality, such as reducing productivity, flattening emotional responses, diminishing a sense of responsibility, and potentially causing addiction not to mention the side effects of stronger psychotropic drugs. Psychotropic drugs are the most commonly prescribed medications worldwide. In the FRG alone, for example, 12 to 15 tons of diazepam are prescribed annually, equating to over a billion tablets."

I was shocked by this information. Of course, psychotropic drugs are sometimes indicated, but in many clinics, their use is excessive. Certainly, a psychological disorder often has a biochemical correlate. However, if a patient is treated solely with psychotropic drugs without simultaneously attempting to reintegrate the patient into their community or family the possible source of the conflict doesn't this amount to merely an organic treatment of a psychosomatic disorder?

I believe that a doctor in Africa who would handle psychotropic drugs as liberally as this would be doing a disservice to the population. Such liberality would be a curse for us Africans!

The success of psychotropic drug marketing and their acceptance by conventional medicine causes me to fear that, before Africa has enough antibiotics to treat its infectious diseases, it will soon be flooded by an excessive number of psychotropic drugs. As a result, we might end up not only with untreated infectious diseases but also with persistent or even medication-induced psychological disorders.

The medical men have shown us that some patients can be treated successfully without psychotropic drugs. It is not necessarily required to have many hours of psychotherapy over months or years.

"The real effectiveness of traditional transcendental medicine largely relies on psychotherapy. The psychotherapeutic neutralization of mental disorders that are exacerbated or intensified by the respective concepts of illness, as well as the psychopathological overlays and negative social consequences of unavoidable diseases, also constitutes a causal therapy from a scientific perspective. That a strengthening of the defense mechanisms and healing tendencies can indeed be achieved through psychotherapy, even in purely somatic' diseases, is an old experience and is proven, among other things, by placebo experiments or miracle-like cures in hypnosis."

Against facts, there are no arguments!

The constant presence of a psychotherapeutic team in the internal medicine-surgical emergency clinic, both day and night, has, among other things, shown that many patients who come in with symptoms of appendicitis or a cardiac attack are actually suffering from anxiety and panic reactions or other emotional problems of various kinds, which can be treated through short-term psychotherapy. This is particularly true for the night hours, when emotional and psychosomatic disorders occur much more frequently.

For many patients, it is often enough to receive a small hint or key word to understand where the conflict might lie. The patient themselves is willing to continue processing their problem and actively find the necessary solution. Isn't this help much more genuine and long-lasting in healing than immediate sedation of the patient? Such treatment also aligns with the expectations of the average African, i.e., that after such treatment, they feel more capable of reintegrating into society and being accepted. Especially when an African is ill, values regarding tradition, family, and their identity as a person and member are strongly present in their consciousness. Any medical or health measure that respects their person, needs, and worldview during treatment will certainly be met with cooperation.

Finally, I would like to quote the reflections of Prof. Dr. Pohl:

"The sick person is a symbol - in them, the fundamental conditions of all human reality are reflected. The medical history is the life history - the subject of medicine is the person, not just a sick organ. Health is not the absence of disorders; health is the strength to live with them.

The concept of health by which contemporary society defines itself is too much about escaping reality and too little about a sense of reality.

Simply having pain is, therefore, not generally considered a disease.

And here it is about more than polymathy and scientific accuracy; mentality, worldview, world image, and, first and foremost, the image of man plays a role."

With that, I come to my next chapter: What is this worldview? To what extent should it be respected without interfering with medical health measures?

Further Reading

1. See Wolf Wimmer, ***Witch Hunt at Universities?*** In: Journal of General Medicine, 56th Year, 1980, Issue 22, p. 1390 ff
2. Josef Neumann, ***Indigenous Medicine and European Medicine in Cameroon***, edited by E. Seidler and Barbro Kuhlo, Freiburg, Hans Ferdinand Schulz Verlag, 1978, p. 198
3. See Josef Neumann, ***Indigenous Medicine and European Medicine in Cameroon***, op. cit., p. 216
4. Djuvanovic and E.P. Mach, A Joint UNICEF/WHO Study, ***Alternative Approaches to Meeting Basic Health Needs in Developing Countries***, 1975, p. 84
5. Paul Diepgen, ***History of Medicine***, Volume 1, Berlin: Walter de Gruyter & Co, 1949, p. 24

6. Hans Joachim Diesfeld, ***Alternative Medical Systems***, In: Curare, Journal of Ethnomedicine and Transcultural Psychiatry, Vol. 3, 1980, p. 131 - 132
7. See Len Holdstock, ***Indigenous Healing in South Africa and the Person-Centered Approach of Carl Rogers***, In: Curare, Journal of Ethnomedicine and Transcultural Psychiatry, Vol. 4, 1981, p. 31 -46
8. See Paul Hinderling, ***Is the Medicine Man a Diviner, Exorcist, ...?*** In: Curare, Vol. 4, 1981, p. 115
9. See Paul Hinderling, op. cit., p. 115
10. See Paul Kapapa, ***The Traditional Healer in Malawi and Zambia***, In: Curare, Vol. 3, 1980, p. 205 ff
11. Hermann Baumann, ***The Peoples of Africa and Their Traditional Cultures***, Wiesbaden, Franz Steiner Verlag, 1975, p. 805
12. Ulf Lind, Disease, ***Healing, and Healing Arts***, edited by H. Schippergers, E. Seidler, and P. Unschuld, Freiburg/Munich: Karl Alber Verlag, 1978, p. 60
13. G. Jansen, ***Doctor-Patient Relationship in an African Tribal Society***, Assen, Van Goncum & Comp. B.V., 1973, p. 142
14. See Djuvanovic and E.P. Mach, ***A joint UNICEF/WHO Study***, op. cit., p. 84
15. Alexander Sturm, ***Basic Concepts of Internal Medicine and Neurology,*** Stuttgart, Gustav Fischer Verlag, 1968, p. 234 ff
16. See Ulf Lind, ***Disease, Healing, and Healing Arts***, op. cit., p. 58
17. See Antonio Scarpa, ***The Revival of Traditional Medicine***, op. cit., p. 37 ff
18. Sebastian Goeppert, ***Medical Psychology***, Volume 2, Rowohlt Taschenbuch Verlag GmbH, 1980 p. 180
19. See Promotion and Development of Traditional Medicine, op. cit., p. 27 ff
20. Richard Kepp and H. J. Stemmier, ***Textbook of Gynecology***, Stuttgart, Georg Thieme Verlag, 1980, p. 300 ff
21. See Paul Diepgen, ***History of Medicine***, op. cit., p. 22
22. See Paul Diepgen, ibid.
23. See Antonio Scarpa, ***The Revival of Traditional Medicine***, op. cit., p. 38
24. See Ulf Lind, Disease, ***Healing***, and Healing Arts, op. cit., p. 57
25. L. Bellak/L. Small, ***Short Psychotherapy and Emergency Psychotherapy***, Frankfurt/M., Suhrkamp Verlag, 1972, p. 25

G. Pfohl, ***The Doctor Between Technology and Healthcare***, In: Med. World, Volume 29, Issue 33, 1978, p. 1296

Notes

[xiii] See J.D. Rosch MD, ***Biology and its Use***. In: International Foundation for Biosocial Development and Human Health, Vol. 2, 1981, p. 12-13

[xiv] John M. Janzen, ***The Quest of Therapy in Lower Zaire***, USA: University of California Press, 1978, p. 61 - 62

[xv] See ***Traditional Medicine in Africa***, In: Series of Technical Reports Afro (WHO), No 1, 1976, p. 5 ff

[xvi] See ***Promotion and Development of Traditional Medicine***, World Health Organization (WHO), No 622, 1978, p. 7 ff

[xvii] See John M. Janzen, ***The Quest of Therapy in Lower Zaire***, op. cit., p. 51 – 52

[xviii] See Djuvanovic and E.P. Mach, A joint UNICEF/WHO Study, op. cit., p. 46 ff

[xix] Erwin Ackerknecht, ***Medicine and Ethnology***, Bern, 1971, p. 93 ff

[xx] See John M. Janzen, ***The Quest of Therapy in Lower Zaire***, op. cit., p. 51

[xxi] See Josef Neumann, ***Indigenous Medicine and European Medicine in Cameroon***, op. cit., p. 46 - 47

[xxii] Ulf Lind, ***Disease, Healing, and Healing Arts***, op. cit., p. 52

[xxiii] See Paul Diepgen, ***History of Medicine***, op. cit., p. 12

[xxiv] Antonio Scarpa, ***The Revival of Traditional Medicine***, In: Curare, Journal of Ethnomedicine and Transcultural Psychiatry, Vol. 3, 1980, p. 31 ff

CHAPTER III

OUR AFRICAN WORLDVIEW

1. Even the Dying Patient Needs a Doctor

Before beginning, I must inform the reader that I do not intend to present the entire worldview here, but rather only a few points that play a role in our understanding of illness and health.

First, I would like to share a personal experience from my internship and use this example to highlight an aspect of our worldview in contrast to the Western one.

Patient X came to the emergency room, and as an intern, I examined him under the supervision of an assistant doctor. This patient later came to the ward where I was interning. From the beginning, I was interested in his treatment and wanted to learn about his fate as a person.

Here is part of the medical history and findings of Patient X, which I documented:

Medical History: Patient X came to us due to persistent coughing. He has had mucous, glassy sputum for more than 4 weeks, with no blood present. He complains of exertional dyspnea and insomnia. His weight has remained constant, although he has no appetite.

Bowel movements, urine: Normal. Otherwise, he has always been healthy.

Social History: Married, 2 children, stable family situation.

Findings: Approximately 1.70 m tall, 65 kg, 44-year-old patient, in moderately good general condition, no signs of distress.

On the left supraclavicular area, a firm, hazelnut-sized, movable lymph node is palpable. Single spider naevi.

Lungs: Breathing sounds reduced on the right lower base. Percussion sound dull on the right lower base.

Pleural effusion on the right lower base.

Heart: Heart sounds clear, no extrasystoles, no additional heart sounds. Heart apex beat: within the mid-clavicular line.

Pulse rate: 100/min, regular, blood pressure 150/80.

Abdomen: Soft abdominal wall, no tenderness to pressure, no resistance palpated. Liver dullness: 13 cm.

Extremities: No varicose veins, no edema. Strongly palpable foot pulses on both sides.

Reflexes: Normal orientation neurological exam.

Psychological: Anxious expression.

Order: Chest X-ray in 2 views, EKG, blood test, electrolytes, blood sugar, urine analysis, sputum culture, Tine test, and admission to the hospital for diagnosis clarification and therapy.

Preliminary Diagnosis: Persistent cough of unclear origin, e.g., tuberculosis, bronchial cancer, bronchopneumonia, etc.

The doctor I was on duty with was satisfied with my medical history and findings for Patient X, and he ordered hospital admission.

The attending physician also ordered the following additional tests:

- Upper abdominal ultrasound
- Abdominal X-ray (overview) in standing position
- Pleural puncture
- Colon contrast enema
- Bone scintigraphy
- Blood culture
- Computer tomography (CT)
- Lymph node biopsy.

The histology report came back with the following findings:

"Decaying lymph nodes of a large cell carcinoma; the tumor is consistent with the clinical suspicion of bronchial carcinoma."

The findings from the native abdominal CT scan are as follows:

"The liver is markedly enlarged. Its cranio-caudal extent in the midclavicular line (MCL) is 15 cm. The liver contains multiple irregularly defined hypodense areas of varying sizes, with a particularly large area located in the dorsal portion of the left liver lobe. Behind the right liver lobe, there is a hypodense layer of fluid-equivalent density, which corresponds to ascites. The spleen and gallbladder are unremarkable. The pancreas is poorly delineated and appears somewhat altered.

The adrenal regions are unremarkable. There is a large hypodense mass at the upper pole of the right kidney. A smaller hypodense mass is noted at the upper pole of the left kidney. Based on density measurements, these masses correspond to cysts."

The patient was informed of these findings. Unfortunately, I was not present during this visit. I asked my attending physician about Patient X and learned that he had left the following note:

"DECLARATION"

Against the advice of the doctor, I am leaving the hospital today at my explicit request and also at my own responsibility. I have been informed by the medical staff about the possible consequences of this decision."

Signature of the doctor Signature of the patient

A week later, the patient returned to us due to increasing dyspnea, weakness, and coughing. After explaining the treatment with cytostasis and its potential side effects and chances of success, the patient agreed to the therapy. A few days later, the attending physician wrote the following to the general practitioner:

"Re: Mr. X,

Date of birth: [date]

Diagnosis: Large-cell bronchial carcinoma.

We started with a polychemotherapy regimen including Platinex X VP 16-213, Adriamycin, Cyclophosphamide, Vincristine, according to the attached scheme. The 8th day of the treatment has been completed, and the next dose of chemotherapy will be administered on the 22nd day of the scheme, so we request readmission on [date] 1978. We discharged Mr. X on [date] 1978 with subjective wellbeing for further treatment under your care.

Therapy suggestions: 2x1 Eusaprim forte for approximately 5 days. Symptomatically, Tricodein capsules may be prescribed. Please check the leukocytes and platelets or the complete blood count once a week."

On [date], 1978, Patient X came in for further cytostatic treatment, and his file documented:

"Large-cell bronchial carcinoma of the right lower lobe with suspected progression under cytostatic treatment.

44-year-old patient now in a significantly reduced general condition. Noticeable blue skin and visible mucous membranes. No edema, no generalized lymph node enlargement.

Diffuse alopecia of the scalp under cytostatic treatment. Otherwise, head unremarkable. Supraclavicular, hard, hazelnut-sized, movable lymph nodes; occasional spider naevi.

Spine not tender to pressure."

The cytostatic treatment continued, and on [date], 1978, we discharged Patient X to home. On [date], 1979, this final report was written:

"Mr. X is now in a significantly worsened general condition compared to the last hospital stay. He was admitted for the continuation of a polychemotherapy cytostatic regimen with Platinex X VP 16-213, Adriamycin, Cyclophosphamide, and Vincristine. In addition to the worsening general condition, the X-ray now showed an abnormal finding in the right basal area, indicating that despite the previous cytostatic therapy, progression of the tumor process must be suspected.

Since the cytostatics administered this time have a different mechanism of action than those previously given, the aforementioned regimen was continued. It should also be mentioned that the patient himself insisted on continuing the cytostatic treatment..."

In 1979, an ultrasound control examination was performed with the following assessment:

<u>"Control sonography from 1979"</u>

Compared to the previous examination, two hypoechoic, rounded areas are now found on the dorsal contour of the left liver lobe, which, given the underlying condition, can be interpreted as tumor necrosis or necrotizing metastases in the context of known large-cell bronchial carcinoma, (see photo documentation) The rest of the livers structural pattern is homogeneous, with no further structural defects.

During the clinical stay of patient X, we visited him daily, just like our other patients with pneumonia, cor pulmonale, cerebral sclerosis, etc. However, with this patient, our questions were particularly focused on the side effects of cytostatics, "Are you suffering from nausea? How is your bowel movement? How is urination? Do you feel particularly weak?"

Later in 1979, our visit was more profound. After the greeting, the attending physician said the following to the patient:

"I spoke with my chief physician, Prof. Dr., who is an expert in oncology, and we discussed your condition. We both believe that we can now discharge you. Despite our aggressive therapy, unfortunately, the course of your illness cannot be positively influenced. We do not know of any other treatment that could help you better. We believe that you would prefer to spend the last time of your life at home with your family rather than being confined to a hospital bed. Why should we continue to torment you with our cytostatics and their side effects when we cannot truly achieve any improvement? Have you had a lot of pain lately? We will try in the next 2-3 days to find the best pain medication for you and then recommend it to your family doctor so he can continue to prescribe it."

"Doctor, how long do I have left to live?" the patient interrupted the attending physician's monologue.

"Mr. X, I cannot tell you this in advance. It could be a few months or even a year, or years. I really don't know. I think it would be even more unpleasant for you to know the exact time. I myself would be very unhappy if I knew in advance that I had to die tomorrow. Of course, you must deal with this problem on your own. Every patient processes their death differently. Some turn to religion, others do not believe in God. How you decide is up to you, but you certainly cannot do this so well in the hospital. But if you really want to stay in the hospital or if we should continue treating you with cytostatics, you are welcome to stay here."

I can't find the right words to describe how I empathized with the loneliness of this patient. It was like a great vacuum between us and him.

A few months later, we were informed by the family doctor that Patient X had passed away at home. This case prompted me to reflect on our African worldview, the doctor, the family, and death.

It seems to me that, in the case of Patient X, as soon as the doctor or doctors made their prognosis, they no longer considered themselves responsible for the patient, so to speak, as if there were no longer a doctor for this patient. One might still ask, will the family doctor continue to be the "doctor" for the patient? Will the doctor-patient relationship be maintained at least with the family doctor?

I recall a lecture in general medicine, where our professor shared how difficult it is to care for a "dying" patient.

"I myself," the professor said, "had a patient with a melanoma. During a home visit, I truly didn't know what to say to the family or the patient. In embarrassment, I took out my stethoscope and, as if by ritual, I told the patient, 'Breathe in deeply and exhale.' I checked the pulse and said at the end: 'Good, here's the medication for pain.' When I repeated the same thing on another visit, and was already at the door, the patient's brother approached me and asked: 'Doctor, have you touched my brother's face and noticed how he reacts to it? That does him so much good.' I turned around, and when I stroked the patient's face, he gave me a friendly and spontaneous smile and said: 'Thank you, doctor, goodbye, see you soon.'"

When discharging Patient X, I wondered what would happen to him next. Wouldn't he become a "burden to his family and his family doctor? He might have been a kind father to his family, but now he is someone who needs pity, and the family must be very careful with him so as not to hurt his feelings in his final moments. Can a patient, therefore, also be lonely in their family?

In this case, I asked myself what limits are placed on the doctor. I was very impressed by the technical examination of Patient X and how his diagnosis was properly made. But I still believe that despite the grim diagnosis, Patient X should have the right to a doctor one who prescribes him more than just painkillers. Just as the patient needs a family that doesn't just pity him, but accepts him as a "whole" person; one who alleviates his loneliness and shares the burden of his fate.

When someone celebrates a party out of joy, they like to see their friends share in the happiness. The same applies when someone is sad. They want their loved ones to be with them, not just passively, but actively. It is a relief, even a joy, to feel that one is embraced by the company of healthy people, even in the final days of life. One would not be surprised to see someone pass away with dignity, smiling as they say goodbye to their family: "It really has been nice with you here in this world. We've had fun together; sometimes I hurt you, but I meant well. Who knows? Maybe we'll meet again."

I believe the concept of a doctor must be broader. For example, when a pregnancy is detected, the doctor essentially becomes the caregiver for both the mother and the unborn child, and they remain the doctor from the early childhood check-ups all the way into old age. The doctor should also be a companion and friend to the dying person.

I am aware that, for the European reader, this may appear to be a utopia. But this is the worldview I know and deeply appreciate, even more so today, especially after experiencing Europe.

I know that recently, even in the West, there has been an effort to improve care for the dying. For example, in the "Hospital Tribune" from February 23, 1982, No. 4, there is an article titled:

"Must one die in a hospital?"

"About 70% of our fellow humans die in hospitals, around 20% in nursing or care homes, and only about 10% at home in their own apartments. However, when asked, up to 92% of the dying people express the desire to die at home. The remaining 8%, who do not have such a wish, are those who no longer have a home. This discrepancy between the needs of the dying and the actual situation makes death in our time often undignified."

In Great Britain, St. Christopher Clinic is internationally known as a "hospice clinic." However, many problems still exist, and there are even "efforts in the USA to pay for foreign assisted dying with a state fee," as was further mentioned in the Hospital Tribune!

It is my belief that where such a worldview already exists, it should be further supported by us doctors, and we must also find our role in such a context. Regarding a worldview that does not sharply distinguish between life, illness, and death, Albert Schweitzer wrote admiringly:

"First, I notice that the natural child is much more 'thoughtful' than we usually assume. Even though it cannot read and write, it has considered many more things than we think.

Conversations that I have had with old natives in my hospital about the last questions of life have deeply moved me. The difference between white and colored, educated and uneducated disappears when you talk with the jungle people about the questions concerning our relationship to ourselves, to others, to the world, and to the Eternal. 'The Negroes are deeper than we are because they don't read newspapers,' a white man said to me recently. There is some truth in this paradox.

The natural child does not fear death; instead, it sees it as something natural. The more medieval form of Christianity, where the fear of judgment is at the forefront, finds much less resonance with him than the more ethical one. To him, Christianity is the moral worldview revealed by Jesus, the teaching of the Kingdom of God and the grace of God.

In the natural man, an ethical rationalist slumbers. He has a natural receptivity to the concept of the Good and what resonates with it in religion. Certainly, Rousseau and the people of the Enlightenment idealized the natural child. But there is some truth in their view of the good and reasonable disposition within him.

One should not think that the worldview of the "Negro" has been described simply by taking a precise inventory of his inherited superstitious beliefs and traditional legal views. He does not turn inward; rather, he is subjected to them. In his being, there is a dim intuition that the understanding of what is good must arise from reflection."

Or as Senghor expresses it:

"But there are no boundaries in Black Africa, not even between life and death. The real only reaches its density, becomes truth, when it breaks through the narrow framework of logical reason, when it spreads into the stretchable vastness of the supernatural.

This means that the Negro-African surrealism is a cosmological naturalism, a supernaturism."

2. Some concepts from our worldview and their implications

I believe I do not need to provide proof to the reader as to why the patient's worldview is important for the doctor. When an African is ill, the first question is, WHY am I sick? Because of the evil eye of my aunt or my mother-in-law? In other words: the African is convinced that every illness has a psychological component that plays a role. The medicine man's first task is to help the patient find the psychological cause of the illness. After that, the patient will actively remove his psychological or social misbehavior and, with the inner peace now achieved, will be receptive to being healed by medication for the "organic part" of the illness.

Is this view of illness and its treatment so foreign to Europeans? I have the impression that recently, in Europe, sick people are also asking, WHY are they sick? In the past, it was a stigma in industrialized countries to suffer from a psychological conflict or psychosomatic illness. But today, with increasing environmental stress, it is becoming more difficult to deny the psychological component of many diseases.

"There have always been psychosomatic illnesses, even if they were less in fashion than they are today."

Or

"In recent years, it has been widely agreed that 30-50% of patients seeking medical help exhibit so-called 'functional disorders.' The cause of these forms of illness should not primarily be attributed to material factors, but to the strong and fitting expression catastrophic experiences. This means that 'tensions,' 'excitations,' and 'fears' arise in the emotional relationships between people, which no longer allow for symptom-free processing. The individual's personal wishes collide so forcefully with prohibitions that conflicts arise, to which the individual's emotional resilience can no longer withstand.

The preferred therapy, therefore, is the attempt to help the patient achieve an emotional correction, to process experiences in a reality-appropriate manner, and to strengthen their ego function. Not only the individual constitution, not only the individual's life fate with its scenarios in which well-known figures appear as actors, but also social, pathological conditions influence human behavior and are reflected in the clinical pictures.

Each of these studies, building on Freud's insights and modern psychology's understanding of the reciprocal influence between organic and psychological processes, sees illness as a manifestation of deep, often hidden behavioral disorders; illnesses express something.' They signal individual and social suffering, misfortune, or wellbeing, and they articulate conflicts that the doctor must decipher and understand in order to facilitate healing."

The last part of the above quote is nothing other than the expectations of an average African towards his doctor or medicine man.

To this worldview, there is also the central concept of "MENSCH" (human), which is translated into most African languages as "NTU" and thus the word BANTU. In everything we do, whether we are healthy or ill, this concept "NTU" - strength = human is very important.

"Building upon grammar ultimately, on language after Abbe Alexis Kagame, Janheinz Jahn discovers, in the Negro-African ontology, force as the very essence of beings, which is expressed through the root "nt" in Bantu. Thus, within the framework of nominal classes, muntu designates "the force endowed with intelligence"; *kintu*, "the forces which... only come into action through the intervention of a Muntu"; *bantu*, "the force that localizes, in time and space, every event"; *kuntu*, "finally... rhe modal force," such as laughter or beauty, for example, which constitute, "in the eyes of the Bantu, authentic forces."

So, it is not precisely having force as an attribute, but being a force as substance, that forms the common quality and, in fact, the identity of beings, since Father Placide Tempels, in translating the "Bantu" thought, posited that "Being IS force." All the great Africanists and primarily the African informants and researchers have confirmed this fundamental principle of African ontology. This could, just as well, be formulated as: "The fabric of matter is energy."

Thus, instead of being separate from one another, distinct and incommunicable, in any case without action on each other, each being-force, each *ntu*, by its natural nature and own movement, can influence another, and all the more easily if the latter is subordinate to it.

The world of forces is, therefore, a system of communicating vessels: a communion of beings among themselves and in Being."

Or in other words:

"The Negro identifies Being with life, more precisely, with life force.

But this force, the foundation of spiritual and moral, therefore immortal life, can only truly be alive and grow if it is embodied in a person, if it is linked with body and breath of life. These two, made of matter, are perishable and dissolve after death.

But man is not alone in the world. One of his similar life forces animates every sentient object, from God to a grain of sand. The Negro has established a strict hierarchy of forces. At the top, a single God, an uncreated creator:

"He, the force itself, who has the force from within himself. He grants existence, substance, and growth to the other forces." Below him come the ancestors, first the founders of the tribes, the "godlike" ones. Then, as one goes down the ladder, the living, who are mostly ordered according to tradition, often by firstborn. Finally, at the end of the ladder, the classes of animals, plants, and minerals, and within each class, the same hierarchy.

Here, the extraordinary position of the human being as a person, as an active being, who can strengthen his existence, in this system,, must be emphasized. For the universe is a closed system of forces, which are individually distinct, but solidaristic. The entire creation is therefore centered around man. To the extent that Being is life force, the ancestors, if they do not want to be non-existent, "completely dead" (as the Bantu expression goes), must dedicate themselves to the reinforcement of the life of the existing, which allows them to take part in it. As for the lesser beings, animals, plants, minerals, they have no other goal in God's plan than to support the deeds of the dead. They are tools, not ends in themselves."

For us Africans, the concept of "HUMAN" as force, energy is of fundamental importance in the context of illness and health. In this context, we come to the term "Witchcraft," which describes the universe as a closed system of forces that, while individually distinct, are solidaristic with one another. The term "Witchcraft" is still superficially understood or completely misunderstood in literature. For example, as M. J. Feld wrote:

"The Akan word usually translated as "witch" is obayifo, meaning a person who is the abode of an evil entity, the obayi. It is believed that covens of witches - numbering usually between ten and twenty under a group leader, hold secret nocturnal meetings in inaccessible places and travel to these gatherings by flying through the air or by riding on antelopes, leopards and owls. The meetings are cannibalistic feasts: the bodies of the witches' victims are cut up, cooked in a pot (the bayseaa) and eaten. The fact that a witch has been demonstrably asleep on her mat throughout the night she is supposed to have spent in feasting, and the fact that the corpse of her victim, slain supposedly by witchcraft, has clearly suffered no cannibalistic ravages, are covered by African dogma. It is the spirit of the witch that leaves her sleeping body and flies to the meeting place. It is not the victim's material body but his vital kra which is eaten by the witches."

These "stories," among others, are familiar to me, but what is the underlying thought?

Witchcraft is primarily interpreted by many researchers as fear-inducing and as a form of empty superstition (see Chapter 1, "Peculiarities of the Medical History in Our Culture"). One could write a book about the phenomenon of witchcraft, and I would go too far if I tried to report on it here. I only want to point out that witchcraft is fundamentally based on the observation that many events, regardless of distance, can have an impact on a person's health or fate. If, as our Bantu philosophy says, everything is force or energy, then what is essential in the relationship between different forces is that they mutually influence one another. Perhaps the following quote may help clarify this; although it is not entirely the same, it can be used as a useful analogy to European thought:

"Caplan spoke of the 'emotional carrier of germs,' meaning that the emotionally charged atmosphere in a family, a small community, a factory, or other defined group situations often largely originates from a single emotionally disturbed person. There are school classes or entire neighborhoods where a single disturbed adolescent creates significant tensions. With timely intervention from appropriately trained teams of psychotherapists, it might be possible to prevent such individuals from infecting the entire group. For preventive measures of this type, two main things are necessary: first, appropriate methods of detection and prediction, and second, short psychotherapeutic procedures for preventive treatment."

Or like:

"Here's an example of how short-term psychotherapy can serve as part of a social psychiatric program for prevention: Hilgard and Newman studied the onset of symptoms in a large number of patients at a psychiatric institution and found, particularly among women, a surprising frequency of a phenomenon they called "anniversary psychosis." A significant percentage of these women became psychotic when their oldest child reached the age at which the patients themselves had lost their mothers. For example, Mrs. Jones had lost her mother at the age of six; her acute psychosis began when her oldest child turned six. This coincidence likely triggered a series of conflicts for Mrs. Jones. One might hypothesize, for instance, that she strongly identified with her daughter and, at this point, experienced significant anger, jealousy, and fear. Another possible hypothesis is that she identified her daughter with her own mother, and that this reversal of psychological positions caused considerable stress for her."

In our understanding, the daughter could be considered a "Witch," just like the "emotional germ carrier" mentioned in the above quote.

The medicine man's task is to recognize this fact and carry out an appropriate treatment. Everything else regarding witchcraft and what is written about it is secondary to this fact. It's like telling a child a story about evil spirits to stimulate their imagination, with the important part being the moral behind it.

However, even more important than the concept of witchcraft, derived from our philosophy of NTU, is the idea of how one becomes healthy. As I mentioned, energy, or activity, is necessary for this.

Unfortunately, this concept is not yet recognized by Western medicine, which could otherwise be used to encourage better cooperation from the population in various health measures or to build positive compliance between doctor and patient. Many European doctors who work or have worked in Africa mistakenly think that many African patients are reluctant to take medication and only do so irregularly. That's why many of these doctors require patients to take their medication in front of them or in front of a nurse or caregiver. Unfortunately, this completely contradicts our worldview of NTU (= force, energy)! The patient wants to feel that they have a chance to actively do something for their health. In other words, the patient wants to be challenged so that their "NTU" can be set in motion.

From the perspective of the Bantu African, therapy means the energy and determination of the patient (and their family) to be healed with the help of the doctor. The medicine man has correctly understood this and supports it. For example, if a doctor prescribes a few aspirin tablets, they would say: "Please take one aspirin in the morning, afternoon, and evening, etc." If the medicine man were to prescribe the same tablets, he would first say: "Please remember that before taking these tablets, you must offer a sacrifice to your ancestors, such as pouring a little soup on the ground. Then take one tablet in the morning, afternoon, and evening." In this way, the patient must do something for themselves, beyond just swallowing the tablets, and they feel proud that they have proven they truly want to get healthy again. Supervision during tablet intake is unnecessary. The following well-known fairy tale in Africa, documented by Tunde Okanlawon from Nigeria in his dissertation, illustrates how the medicine man can demand this activity (NTU) from his patient.

Once upon a time, there was a woman who was not leading a happy marriage. It seemed to her that everything she did annoyed her husband. She thought a lot about this. Sometimes she believed it was because other women were in love with her husband, and that he enjoyed this. Sometimes she thought it was because she associated with bad people whom her husband couldn't stand. But instead of working on improving her relationship with her husband, she began to behave poorly in order to take revenge on him. She no longer spoke a word to him, even when he was home all day. After some time, she even refused to cook for him and told him to go to his concubines and eat there. She believed her husband had no time for her because he loved other women outside of their marriage. After watching this patiently for a while, her husband decided to take revenge in his own way and began to show her less affection. He became reluctant to return home from work in the afternoons and spent most of his time with his friends. His wife didn't know what to do. After a while, she could no longer stand it, because she felt her husband wanted to leave her.

One day, she went to a medicine man to inquire about what she could do to make her husband stay at home and be kind to her again. The medicine man realized from her story that the woman was jealous and that she mainly lacked patience. He asked her if she was willing to follow his advice, and she agreed. Then, the medicine man asked her to bring him lion's milk so that he could mix a medicine for her. This medicine was supposed to have the power to make both husband and wife fall deeply in love with each other. She looked up to the sky, thinking it over, and desperately asked herself, "Where will I find lion's milk?" But she was determined to obtain the milk, for her marriage was on the verge of falling apart.

"The child is not that shapeless and crying larva that keeps parents awake at night. For Black African parents raise their children in an atmosphere of tenderness and freedom. This 'self-education is not irresponsibility, but vigilant love. It is maintained until the reasonable age when the boy or girl must undergo the harsh trials of initiation ceremonies. From them, a complete man or a complete woman emerges, capable of defying life. Thus, the Black African family is not only turned towards the past, from whose fertile traditions it draws, but also towards the future; more precisely, the past prepares the future.

The woman occupies the first place in Black Africa - she certainly did, as the influence of the Arab-Berbers, later of Europeans, and thus the influence of nomadic civilizations, has not ceased to diminish her position. This position can be explained by the agricultural nature of the Black world. However, this explanation, though correct, is not enough. How liberally has consciousness here transformed an economic-social reality into a myth. The woman, as the 'continuing' member of the family and the giver of life, has been appointed the source of life force and the guardian of the house, which means the repository of the past and the guarantor for the future of the clan."

The importance of family in African culture cannot be emphasized enough. First, I would like to report on a case I experienced here in Germany.

Dr. jur. X, 45 years old, survived his second heart attack and was transferred from the intensive care unit to our internal medicine department. During the first visit, he impatiently and firmly asked when he could go home. He had a business to run, and at that moment, nothing could proceed without him. Moreover, he had important appointments to attend.

Patient Dr. jur. X refused a heart catheterization because it would mean additional time loss. At our request, his wife tried to convince him to stay in the hospital for at least another 4 weeks.

The suggestion from his wife that his father's brother, also a successful lawyer, could temporarily represent him almost led to a divorce.

In Africa, Dr. jur. X would not have been able to make this decision alone. His wife and other important family members had the right, based on medical advice, to continue assigning him the role of patient (see Chapter 1).

Indeed, how many patients in industrialized countries are eager to go home because they fear being viewed as failures by their families and acquaintances, as fathers, businesspeople, etc.?

Even after discharge, when the family assigns the patient the role of patient, the doctor can expect that the recommended restrictions and/or exercises will be followed. This not only ensures better compliance but also minimizes the chances of the patient developing feelings of inferiority because they no longer have to meet their previous performance standards.

Johannes Siegrist et al. write in an extensive medical sociological case-control study (on social stress and heart attack), which was conducted over several years with the support of the German Research Foundation, the following:

"Our research concept is based on three central premises:

There are specific emotional and social stressors that are pathogenetically significant for the premature onset of a heart attack.

These stressors act at least partially independently of the known risk factors for heart attacks and therefore at least partially independently of the process of arteriosclerosis.

The mechanisms that have been assumed, and which have primarily been demonstrated in animal experiments, between central nervous excitations (sympathetic activation), neurohormonal and cardiovascular reactions, and the somatic conditions that can lead to a heart attack (e.g., coronary spasms), are fundamentally detectable in humans as well.

We believe it is essential to distinguish four levels of a process: namely, the risk constellations experienced and processed by the individual, the somatic precursors that arise from long-term recurring central nervous excitations (in the sense of Weiner's bias concept), the pathogenic mechanisms in the strict sense, and finally, the clinical manifestation of the disease."

Postulated Connections in the Research Project

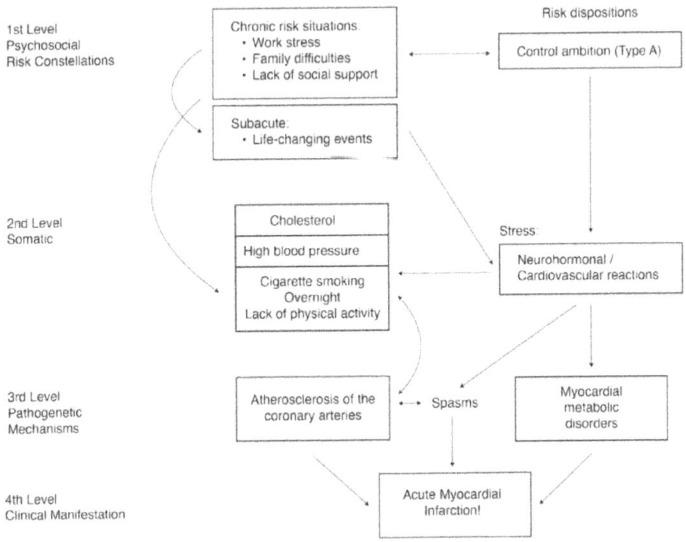

Figure 1. Alter Johannes Siegrist, 1980

If one takes the "postulated connections" seriously, it becomes clear that the assignment or liberation of a patient from their illness role by the African family (and the entire extended family) leads to a significant reduction in risk situations and risk dispositions (see the1st level of Figure 1). As a result, some standard risk factors, i.e., some somatic precursors of a myocardial infarction, were also reduced. Even if the clinical manifestation (4th level of Figure 1) had occurred, the African support role remained of great importance.

"Individuals with strongly developed control ambitions (- risk disposition) are more likely than individuals with average or weak control ambitions to unrealistically assess demanding situations and/or put themselves in situations characterized by a discrepancy between the demands and their ability to cope.

Psychosocial risk factors during the premorbid phase influence the rehabilitation process after a first heart attack: those who died from a recurrent heart attack were more highly burdened than those who survived."

The advantage of our family structures is not only evident in the example of the research project by Siegrist et al. with heart attack patients, but also in many other health conditions. I agree with Prof. Dr. Jean Delacretaz when he says:

"In conclusion, while it is true that the individual is responsible for their health and that anything that tends to take away this responsibility is harmful, it is equally true that the individual cannot bear the burden of their illness alone."

The ideology of the autonomy of the patient is one aspect of contemporary romanticism.

By claiming that one can do without medicine, the romantic ideology isolates the patient, burdens them with a responsibility that crushes them, and removes the recourse to those who can truly help them. This is the second barbarism "generation" in Europe and America. I do not mean to say that everything about the initiation ceremonies was positive (for example, I have a similarly critical opinion about female circumcision as Dr. Fadallah from Sudan in his dissertation "Female Circumcision in the Democratic Republic of Sudan - Hamid Fadallah, Dissertation from 21.8.75, at the Medical Faculty of the University of Berlin").

3. Some Brief Thoughts on the Patient's Psyche and the Apparatuses of Modern Medicine

I believe that in conventional medicine, the psychological aspects of a disease are still underestimated. It is good that technology and its apparatuses have developed diagnostics, treatments, etc., to such an extent (and continue to develop). However, the pure application of technology only brings modest success, as seen, for example, in cancer research: the success of treating advanced malignancies is still unsatisfactory to this day. One is increasingly coming to the conclusion that immunology, endocrinology, and the environment are connected to the development of cancer and its progression. But should this not also inevitably bring the psyche into focus? From our worldview, an affirmative answer would be self-evident.

Gosslar writes:

"Changes in the social environment, emotions, and mood states, such as pain, shock, excitement, as further elaborated, can simultaneously manifest in behavior and somatic processes, with the assumption that all emotional tensions have a material equivalent, which is expressed in hormonal, immunological, biochemical, and other changes. As with Bahnson, who, in explaining his theory of the complementarity of physiological and psychological regression, relies on the general schema of Rakoff (1966), the hypothalamus, as the central control center of the diencephalon, plays an important role in this context: 'From there, indirect hormonal impulses are sent via the pituitary, but also direct nerve impulses to the adrenal glands. In response, they release catecholamines (adrenaline, noradrenaline) and corticosteroids, which in turn influence the bloodstream and immune reactions. This feedback loop between the diencephalon, pituitary, and adrenal glands also involves the gonads and thymus. In the thymus, lymphocytes receive their original programming. Amkraut & Solomon (1975) and Vester (1973) observed in this context that the self-produced antibodies of thymus-derived lymphocytes are responsible for defending against oncogenic viruses and transplanted tumor cells.

The fact that this (monistic) concept of disease development, also in the field of oncology, represents a possible point of approach is supported not least by psychosomatic-oncological animal experiments, primarily from the Soviet school.

These animal experiments have led to two main results: on one hand, an acceleration, and on the other hand, a retardation of tumor growth. The experimental investigations are mostly based on the establishment of conditioned reflexes in animals, which bear some resemblance to the neuroses observed in humans (so-called experimental neuroses).

For example, Petrova (1946) was able to show that experimentally neurotic dogs developed various skin conditions, furunculosis, and chronic ulcerations over time. When these dogs were exposed to chronic stress for several years, they also developed various benign and malignant tumors.

Other experiments on dogs that were permanently traumatized led, after 1 1/2 to 2 years of exposure, to precancerous skin changes upon the application of tar. Papillomas appeared, growing rapidly and spreading to untreated skin areas. In contrast, the control dogs that were treated with tar but were not psychologically stressed also developed papillomas, but they quickly regressed."

In other words, the psyche of the patient - even in the case of cancer patients - can play a significant role. Could one not achieve more success with scientifically proven cancer treatments if formal psychological support were offered to the patient simultaneously? The prospect of conducting such a controlled study fascinated me. Not only because of my firm belief that it would lead to a significant difference in survival time and quality between the control group (i.e., the current classic cancer treatment without formal psychological treatment) and the patients (who would receive formal psychotherapeutic treatment in addition to chemotherapy and/or radiation or surgery), but also because I share this view with Prof. Dr. J. Delacretaz:

"Until the day, probably a distant one, when medicine can cure chronic diseases, it is psychological support that often remains the most essential thing we can offer to those affected. Again, doctors are poorly prepared and often unwilling to provide this kind of support... The only fundamental risk it faces is that it believes that science is medicine, whereas it is only its precious and indispensable servant: the scientistic ideology turns man into a machine; it is the first barbarism that threatens medicine."

I cannot emphasize enough when I say that in our worldview, the psychological "self" is just as central to the concept of health as the body (the organism). I have intentionally connected this worldview with today's increasing health conditions, such as heart attacks, cancer, etc., and I believe these perspectives should be maintained precisely in those contexts. The question now is, what kind of medical history and what kind of conversation creates a good doctor-patient relationship in line with this view of ours?

Further Reading

1. Albert Schweitzer, ***Self-Testimonies***, Munich, C.H. Beck Publishing, 1967, p. 190
2. Leopold Senghor, ***Negritude and Humanism***, Diisseldorf/Koln, Eugen Diedrichs Publishing, 1967, p. 184
3. Jean Delacretaz, ***Medicine Between Two Barbarisms***, Switzerland, Cahiers de la Renaissance, 1979, p. 56
4. Alexander Mitscherlich, ***Disease as Conflict***, Frankfurt/M, Suhrkamp Publishing, 1971, p. 13 ff
5. Leopold Senghor, ***Negritude and the Civilization of the Universal***, Paris, Editions du Seuil, 1974, p. 219
6. Cf. Leopold Senghor, ***Negritude and Humanism***, op. cit., p. 158
7. ibid.
8. MJ. Field, ***Search for Security***, USA, Northwestern University Press, 1962, p. 35
9. L. Beliak and L. Small, **Brief Psychotherapy and Emergency Psychotherapy**, Frankfurt/M, Suhrkamp Publishing, 1972, p. 24
10. Cf. L. Beliak and L. Small, op. cit., p. 23
11. Tunde Okanlawon, **Nigerian Oral Tradition and European Myth Theory**, Frankfurt/M., Peter Lang Publishing, 1977, p. 358
12. Cf. Leopold Senghor, **Negritude and Humanism**, op. cit., p. 208 ff
13. Johannes Siegrist, ***Social Strain and Heart Attack: A Medical Sociological Case-Control Study***, Stuttgart, Enke, 1980, p. 27 ff
    a. Johannes Siegrist, ***Social Strain and Heart Attack***, op. cit., p.29
14. Cf. Jean Delacretaz, ***Medicine Between Two Barbarisms***, op. cit., P- 71
15. J. Dannholz, ***Under the Spell of Belief in Spirits***, Leipzig, Evangelical Lutheran Mission Publishing, 1916, p. 56
16. Leopold Senghor, ***Freedom, Negritude, and the Civilization of the Universal***, Paris, Editions du Seuil, 1977, p. 225
17. Hermann Baumann, ***The Peoples of Africa and Their Traditional Cultures***, Wiesbaden, Franz Steiner Publishing, 1975, p. 43 ff
18. Helmut Gosslar, ***Research on the Cancer Personality***, Frankfurt/M., Fischer Rita Publishing, 1980, p. 37 ff
19. Cf. Jean Delacretaz, ***Medicine Between Two Barbarisms***, op. cit., p. 56

CHAPTER IV

CONNECTION BETWEEN MEDICAL HISTORY AND THE LIFE WORLD OF THE AFRICAN PATIENT

In this chapter, I will attempt to show how a doctor trained in Western medicine can take a medical history from the average African patient, which allows for a good doctor-patient relationship in Africa. The main focus is on how a doctor can move from the patient's reference system to that of Western medicine.

"On the other hand, how can one write about the doctor-patient relationship in Africa without mentioning some pressing issues in the healthcare system that also require this relationship to be confronted?"

The previous chapters have outlined the particularities of the African patient's life world. Here, I would like to explicitly emphasize again that it was never my goal, nor is it now, to support superstition or further propagate mythology quite the opposite. But I am aware that merely banning the traditional healer, as was practiced during colonial times and adopted in many other African countries (cf. Chapter II), without a genuine engagement with the advantages and/or disadvantages, will ultimately lead to no long-term results.

"A recent painstaking investigation of traditional healers and diviners among the Zaramo population of Dar es Salaam has demonstrated that in the capital city of the country, with its relatively high concentration of modernized medical facilities and easy access by public transportation, about 700 full-time traditional diviner healers are practicing medicine using traditional healing methods.... Healing of hurts and illnesses was the predominant activity. ...

Some 4,000 people are treated daily for illness by traditional healers in Dar es Salaam."[xxv] I fully agree with Prof. Dr. Goeppert, who says:

"The doctor has always had the task of enlightenment, with the goal of freeing the relationship between man and health and illness from prevailing myths, and for example, seeing health not only abstractly as freedom from disease, but also taking into account the personal characteristics of his patients as the individual ability and willingness of each person to cope with disabilities, illness, suffering, and pain."[xxvi]

However, for this to happen, the doctor must be somewhat enlightened about the patient themselves. Only then can they speak the same "language" and communicate on the patient's level.

1. The Similarity Between Carl Rogers' Client-Centered Therapy and the Communication of the Medicine Man

During my medical studies, I often wondered or tried to figure out which type of anamnesis could be roughly equated with that of the medicine man. However, when I attended psychotherapy lectures, I suddenly realized that Carl Rogers' "client-centered therapy" had many similarities with the anamnesis of the medicine man. This prompted me to learn more about Rogers' life, interests, and theories, to possibly understand to what extent these similarities actually exist. During my research, I came across an article by Len Holdstock. Due to his friendship and personal collaboration with Rogers, Len Holdstock was able to learn about Rogers' love for nature and his interest in helping others, which were decisive factors in the development of his "client-centered therapy." Len Holdstock concluded that Rogers' therapy is very similar to the communication used by medicine men in Southern Africa.

One might ask, how is an anamnesis a form of therapy? For Africans, an anamnesis is also something mystical (see Chapter I). At the beginning of the conversation, the patient almost impatiently seeks a hint of something magical from the doctor. This is exactly what Albert Schweitzer admired when he noted that his patients only trusted him once they sensed this "magic" in him:

"Now I believe that this is a true doctor!" a heart-sick woman recently exclaimed to Joseph. "He knows that I often can't breathe at night and have swollen feet, and I didn't tell him anything about it, and he didn't even look at my feet."

It's as if the African would take Hippocrates' demand literally: "The doctor should say what has happened before, recognize what is happening now, and predict what will happen in the future."

For the African, the conversation with the doctor is not only the source of trust, but the conversation the word also holds a special place in the worldview. Senghor has written about this and, for example, cites an African poet, Komo-Dibi, to emphasize this point: "The word is everything... It heals or kills, nothing else."

Isn't the "word" to be understood as the first principle? Or as Senghor expresses it: "It (the word) is the ontological fabric of the universe. From this, it follows that the three words Being, Force, and Word are synonymous." If we now remember the importance of the concept of "Being, Force (Ntu)" in the African view of healing (see Chapter III), we see that the conversation with the doctor is on a higher level than a simple "anamnesis" yes, it is an essential part of the therapy, i.e., a "talk therapy."

Now I would like to present some characteristics of the conversation of the traditional healer that are similar to Carl Rogers' client-centered therapy and, as a consequence, attempt to highlight approaches to addressing the health issues in Africa. (However, there are also differences between the two, which cannot be addressed here.)

Len Holdstock discovered that both the traditional healer and C. Rogers recognized that for a good therapist or doctor, not only intelligence but also emotions and feelings are of equal importance.

"Even though Rogers has stated repeatedly since the fifties that we are much wiser than our intellect, very few people in the helping professions and academic world have really pondered the meaning of these words. Gendlin (1973) has been one of the few who elaborated on this key concept in the Person-Centered theory. Bodily wisdom has also been described as organismic sensing, ongoing psychophysiological flow or organismic experiencing. It is the referent to which the individual can and must turn for guidance in understanding himself and in directing his behavior. Without this ongoing psychophysiological flow, it is difficult to develop a concept of self which can withstand the pressure extorted by other people to mold the individual in terms of their expectations. The people of sub-Sahara Africa generally, and the indigenous healers specifically, have been especially strong in their bodily wisdom. Senghor, the poet president of Senegal, expressed it as follows: 'Classical Europe presents us with a civilization of discursive reason; Classical Africa with a civilization of intuitive reason'."

Carl Rogers writes:

"In 1940, I attempted to bring about a shift in the policy of therapy, as I would now call it. Describing an emerging trend, I stated: 'This newer approach differs from the older one in that it has a fundamentally different goal. It directly aims at the greater independence and integration of the individual, rather than hoping that these results will occur when the counselor helps with solving the problem. The individual is the focus, not the problem.'

Over the years, the view I tentatively presented in 1940 has been expanded, deepened, and reinforced through clinical experiences as well as research findings. It became known as client-centered psychotherapy, and in the years since, it has been supported by more empirical studies than any other therapeutic approach.

As an attitude, it has increasingly been recognized, but it must still be acquired step by step to be convinced of its validity. I recently referred to it as the gradually developed and tested hypothesis that the individual carries within themselves an enormous potential for self-awareness and for changing their self-concept, attitudes, and self-determined behavior and that this potential could be released if only we manage to create a definable climate of necessary psychological attitudes.'

What psychological climate is suitable for optimally unlocking the individual's ability to understand and master their life? For such a growth-promoting climate, three conditions are necessary, whether it concerns the relationship between therapist and client, parent and child, group leader and group, teacher and students, administrator and employees it essentially applies to any situation where personal experience is the goal.

The first condition is related to authenticity and genuineness: congruence. The more the therapist is themselves in the relationship and does not hide behind a professional mask or personal facade, the greater the likelihood that the client will change and unfold in a constructive way. This means that the therapist openly expresses the feelings and attitudes that move them in the moment.

What does this mean in practice? It means that when the client feels pain or sorrow, the therapist responds with feelings of warmth, compassion, or understanding. At other moments in the relationship, the therapist may also feel boredom, anger, or even fear of a destructive client. The more the therapist becomes aware of these feelings and is able to experience and express them, whether positive or negative the greater the likelihood that they will be able to help the client. It is the feelings and attitudes that help the other when shared, not opinions or judgments about the other.

The therapist can only be congruent and thus helpful to the extent that they express the feelings they experience. To the degree that the therapist perceives, internalizes, becomes aware of, and expresses what is going on inside them, they will be able to encourage the development of the client.

From the perspective of interpersonal politics, this first element of the relationship congruence creates a maximum space for both the client and the therapist, where they can be themselves. The therapist essentially expresses: "Here I am, as I am."

The above quote not only aligns with the basic attitude of the shaman, but also with the experience most Africans have in their childhood upbringing. In most patriarchal African families, the upbringing generally takes place, as Parin observed among the Dogon, in the following way:

The development of the group self can be traced back to relatively tension-free, identificatory relationships that are established in childhood and adolescence, preferably with same-sex peers in "horizontal" groups. When these relationships are neither disturbed by frustration nor aggression, and when certain "oral" ego characteristics remain, the adult is repeatedly ready to enter into such satisfying relationships. If there are communities or groups in a social situation where, due to their structure and the particular psychology of their members, mutual fraternal or sisterly identifications are possible, the group self is a guarantee for good social adjustment (e.g., in the Dogon village).

By "group self," we mean a specific mode of functioning and a set of particular ego functions, manifestations of the group self, which depend on the participation of a group of people to be sufficient and to remain so. The group must have a certain structure, and its members must respond in a particular way; their emotional readiness and/or ability to assume certain roles is the prerequisite for the group self to function. These ego functions are based on the acquired willingness of the ego to enter into specific identificatory relationships. The group self is, therefore, not a fundamentally different psychic structure from the described ego, nor is it an additional one, as if there were a separate, distinct ego and also a group self.

It is relationships with same-sex peers (peer groups, brotherhoods, various gangs, youth groups, and fraternities) that most easily allow for such identifications. The hierarchical or, sociologically speaking, vertical group organization is counterposed by a parity based, horizontal one. In this, such tension-free identifications can occur, provided the group has sufficiently maternal, nurturing, and breastfeeding behaviors, and is not disturbed too much by rivalry aggression, etc., to allow a temporary "oral regression." When there is a balance in childhood and adolescence between vertical groups of people (following the obligatory vertical pattern of the age-hierarchical family) and horizontal ones, or rather a harmonious alternation between the two, a well-functioning group self is formed, which facilitates later social adjustment to corresponding groups.

In our society, many groups are only seemingly horizontally organized, but in terms of their psychological effect, they exhibit a hierarchical structure. In the Scouts, for example, leadership hierarchy and ideology, or in our schools, the competition-based pressure for performance and the resulting rivalry, outweigh the horizontal age structure of the groups. In these institutions, identification with the aggressor generally occurs, but not a group self.

In our culture, this happens when the nurturing parents step back as individuals in relation to the environment they represent and instead offer the child values or ideologies that are not their own, which may not even guide their behavior or that they themselves fail or fear. If this occurs during critical phases, the inner conflict becomes a lasting acquisition.

Particularly the passive submission to the failing primary figure in the Oedipal conflict seems to be such a sensitive phase, especially when strong feelings of abandonment, the feeling of not being loved, or a deficit in the narcissistic investment of the self-result from the pre-Oedipal development.

Special effects:

We have traced the exemplary sense of community that exists in the traditional Dogon village to an expressed group self. This is developed in a "maternal" group, into which the child enters at the age of four, immediately after a prolonged period of nurturing and symbiotic togetherness with their mother. The group self is strengthened and renewed during adolescence and later in the life of the adult in similarly organized groups consisting of similarly socialized, same-sex, and same-age "peers." It is logical to achieve an education toward better social behavior, which some utopian educational models aim for, by giving children and adolescents the opportunity to form a group self.

This means that the first condition or premise of C. Rogers is nothing other than a situation familiar to the African since birth.

Also, consider what Rogers writes about education:

"The approach to education that we wish to describe does not aim at these goals, but represents an attempt to find a method that can achieve what is called a democratic goal. Whether this goal is appropriate for our current culture is a question that the reader must decide for themselves.

We cannot directly teach another person something; we can only promote their learning.

You can lead the horse to water, but it must drink on its own. However, most teachers operationally ignore this fundamental hypothesis.

If teachers accept students as they are, allow them to express their feelings and attitudes without condemnation or judgment, plan learning activities with them rather than for them, and create an atmosphere in the classroom that is relatively free from emotional pressure and tension, the results are different from when these conditions are not present. These results seem to move toward a democratic goal.

Senghor has also frequently spoken about the role of feeling or emotion in the African:

"It has often been said: The Negro is a person of nature. He is a sensual being, a creature with open senses, without a mediator between subject and object; he is both subject and object at once. He consists first and foremost of sounds, scents, rhythms, forms, and colors; he is rhythm before he is eye, as the European white is eye. He hears more than he sees: he feels. For within himself, in his flesh, he receives and perceives the radiations that every being emits. Set into vibration, he responds to the call and surrenders himself, moving from subject to object, from. I to You on the waves of the Other.

This does not mean that the Negro is devoid of reason, as some have tried to persuade me. But his reason is not deductive; it is synthetic. It is not antagonistic but sympathetic. This is simply another form of knowledge. The Negro's reason does not impoverish things, does not rob them of juice and strength to press them into rigid schemas. It slips into the veins of things, assumes all their forms, in order to immerse itself in the living heart of reality. White reason is analytical for the sake of utility, while Negro reason is intuitive out of empathy.

Hence, the sensitivity of the Black, the power of his emotion. For what grips the Negro is less the appearance of the object than its deeper reality, its higher reality; less its sign than its meaning."

The emphasis is placed on the meaning, the interpretation, which is no longer a practical but a moral and mystical interpretation of reality, thus a symbol. It is also not without interest that contemporary scholars emphasize the primacy of intuitive knowledge through sympathy: "The most beautiful emotion we can experience," writes Einstein, "is the mystical emotion. In it lies the seed of all art and all true science."

C. Rogers adds:

"When the child begins to use its limbs to explore its new environment while lying on the mother's belly, touch becomes a means of communication. Hands preferably those of the mother gently embrace the child or rhythmically stroke its back, reminding it of the familiar inner rhythm. These touches assure the child: We are both still here; we are both alive."

One could extend this analogy further and say: If a doctor, who is naturally and genuinely in touch with his feelings, meets an African patient, he could awaken in him the ancient feelings of security from childhood, thus winning the patient's trust.

Rogers adds more important points of his theory:

"The second attitude that proves essential for the emergence of a climate of change is acceptance, empathy, or appreciation unconditional positive regard. This means that therapeutic development or change is more likely when the therapist has a positive, accepting attitude toward what the client is at this moment.

It is a non-possessive form of regard. The therapist offers the client comprehensive, unconditional appreciation.

The power over his own life remains entirely in the hands of the client. An atmosphere of security is created, not one of coercion."

The same can be experienced with the medicine man. For him, there is no report from a patient that could be considered nonsensical or irrelevant. In this regard, I sought in conventional medicine for an attitude that I could summarize as follows: No matter what apparent incongruity exists between complaints and clinical symptoms; no matter what discrepancy there is between the medical history and findings, the doctor must take the patient's complaint fully seriously and attempt to process it from the patient's perspective, while the doctor must translate the complaints into his system (conventional medicine). This important point will be explained further later in this chapter using concrete examples of medical history and conversation.

Len Holdstock recognized Rogers' "second attitude" in the medicine man as well and wrote:

"It is basically so simple to develop to our full potential. We just have to BE ourselves and KNOW ourselves. In being ourselves we are like no other in the world. Simply being ourselves is our greatest potential. It sounds the easiest thing in the world to be yourself, but it is in fact, extremely difficult. As some-one has said, "To be nobody but yourself in a world which is doing its best, night and day, to make you everybody else, means to fight the hardest battle any human being can fight, and never stops fighting." The opportunity for such an experience is all too rare in an educational and societal structure which consistently bombards us with the message that we are not worthwhile unless we believe in ways which others consider are important for us to follow. The basic trust in the potential of the person, in the dignity and worth of the individual, has earned Rogers the distinction of being described as "one of the most important social revolutionaries of our time". Empowering the person in this way has had some far-reaching implications not only in the helping professions, but also in politics. As in so many other instances, indigenous healing also exhibits striking similarities with the Person-Centered approach in regard to the trust in the potential of the person."

The last point Rogers makes is:

"The third beneficial aspect of the relationship is empathic understanding. This means that the therapist accurately senses the feelings and personal meanings experienced by the client and communicates this understanding to the client. In the most favorable case, the therapist is so deeply immersed in the private world of the other person that they can clarify not only the meanings of which

Gathering, table, or table d'hôte. This immediately brings to mind a small incident that concluded the evening yesterday.

A second association to table d'hôte: A few weeks ago, at a guesthouse table in a Tyrolean Mountain resort, I was quite annoyed with my wife for not being reserved enough toward some neighbors with whom I absolutely did not wish to engage. I asked her to focus more on me than on the strangers. That is, as if I were being neglected at the table d'hôte. Now I also notice the contrast between my wife's behavior at that table and that of Mrs. E.L. in the dream, who turns completely toward me.

Further: I now realize that the dream event is a reproduction of a small scene that occurred quite similarly between my wife and me during the time of our secret courtship. The affection under the tablecloth was a response to a serious courting letter. However, in the dream, my wife is replaced by the stranger E.L."

Len Holdstock, on the other hand, observes:

"The ancestors manifest themselves during waking in the form of visions and voices or in sleep through dreams. What people in the Western world would call hallucinations and delusions are extremely common among the indigenous healers of Southern Africa. These "delusions" guide the healers in their own lives and in their training and treatment of others. Quite recently, Rogers has had intimate contact with experiences of this nature.

In a privately circulated manuscript relating events during the last few months before the death of his wife, Helen, Rogers accounts several of her Spiritual experiences which I would like to construe as visitations by the ancestors. Rogers believes that Helen's gradual acceptance of the validity of her spiritual experience facilitated her acceptance of death as a release from the physical agony which she had been experiencing for so many years.

Dreaming and the discussion of dreams become part of the daily routine training. It is believed that "dreaming is thinking with your heart". Gelfand, a psychiatrist who has extensive associations with the Shona indigenous healers of Rhodesia, regard the claim of diviners to learn through dreams as a method of thought, as a 'utilization of the subconscious mind', for which they are ideally suited "having been born into the culture'."

The life of an African villager is still marked by many taboos. He cannot easily express his anger and disappointments toward older relatives (a vertical group of people). His psyche transforms his consciousness into a form of "symbolic thinking" and fantasy, akin to a dream, similar to Freud's work on dream processes and displacement. The medicine man serves as a kind of built-in valve mechanism; the patient can unburden all their fears and worries to him and fully express themselves in the process.

Thus, it may happen that the medicine man asks the patient: "Did you see a stone on the path?" From the patient's affirmative response, the medicine man "deciphers" the underlying conflicts. Many ethnomedicine practitioners comment on this: "Of course, if the patient came along a path covered with stones, they must have seen a stone. So, the stone and the resolution of the conflict are entirely unrelated."

Interestingly, the explanation is different: the stone represents a symbol. The medicine man's task is to observe the expressions, emotional tensions, and gestures the patient uses to describe the "stone." It is, as Freud says:

"I can describe this fact as follows: During the dreamwork, the psychic intensity transitions from the thoughts and ideas to which it rightfully belongs to others that, in my judgment, have no claim to such emphasis. No other process contributes as much to concealing the meaning of the dream and obscuring the connection between dream content and dream thoughts. During this process, which I want to call dream displacement, I also observe the psychic intensity, significance, or affectivity of thoughts transforming into sensory vividness. The most distinct part of the dream content seems to me immediately to be the most important; yet, I can often recognize the most direct descendant of the essential dream thought in an unclear dream element."

Thus, it may happen that the medicine man ultimately explains that the "stone" represents the patient's father. The father stands in the way, preventing him from marrying a girl from another tribe. The medicine man then gives appropriate advice on how to "remove" this "stone" from the path, and so on. The crucial point here is not only the ability to correctly interpret the symbol "stone" within the cultural context but also a deep empathy that relaxes the patient and allows them to express all their thoughts about the stone (father) "without intention or criticism."

I have already mentioned that the life of the medicine man, as well as the life of the African in general, is accompanied by many emotions. This benefits the medicine man in his empathy.

"When one grows up with many emotions, one does not need to learn much to be more empathetic."

Many ethnomedical practitioners focus on the rites (listening, dancing, discussion, etc.) of the medicine man. He uses objects in his ceremonies, such as animal tails and various small stones. But all this serves only to stimulate the imagination of the patient their state of consciousness and their "mystical feelings." One should not be distracted by these accompanying circumstances, as the focus is more on the effect.

"Paracelsus, that great proponent of mysticism," the same author adds, "was evidently not in doubt about the efficacy of amulets and similar objects when he wrote the following insightful remark:

"It is indifferent whether you believe in something real or something false; it will have the same effect on you. If I believe in a statue of Saint Peter as I would believe in the saint himself, the statue will have the same effect on me as Saint Peter, except that this is superstition. It is always only faith that works these wonders, and whether it pertains to something real or something false, its magical power remains the same."

2. Bridging Traditional African Belief Systems and Modern Medicine

After analyzing the similarities between Rogerian talk therapy and the practices of the traditional medicine man, the question remains: How could these approaches be concretely applied? The following is an authentic example recounted by a doctor who worked as a development aid worker:

A woman, the mother of three children, came to the clinic and claimed that she had been pregnant for thirteen months. Everything had been fine up until the third or fourth month of her pregnancy. However, during this time, her mother-in-law visited, and from that point on, her pregnancy had gone poorly. The mother-in-law had never approved of the marriage in the first place. The woman emphasized that she felt very ill.

The doctor asked the patient if she was aware that an average pregnancy typically lasts nine months.

"Of course," she replied, "but it is well known in our community that if a woman is bewitched, her pregnancy can last up to three years. However, this kind of bewitchment is so dangerous that the woman often dies as a result. If she does survive, she will never have another child in her life. I am scared."

How would one further gather a case history like this?

The simplest approach might be to inform the woman, as mentioned earlier, that pregnancy typically lasts nine months. Retrospectively, she could now be convinced that she is not in her 13th month of pregnancy and likely never was. The issue with her mother-in-law could be dismissed as mere superstition without clinical significance (Perhaps tranquilizers could also be prescribed.)

In this way, the doctor would be genuine. He should not dismiss the patient as simply ignorant but instead offer her an opportunity for dialogue. How else could he aim for a good doctor-patient relationship? The doctor might briefly talk about the mother-in-law and recommend that the patient be kinder to her. This is not about psychotherapy but about an attempt at empathy and warmth. The patient will feel taken seriously and respected in her self-worth. I believe this could create the possibility for a genuine relationship.

I understand that such a model of conversation may be difficult to follow in other situations and with different medical conditions. However, the attempt must be made, along with striving for empathy toward the patient.

Let us return to the issues I mentioned in Chapter 1. A certain doctor had intensively studied the doctor-patient relationship in Africa, unfortunately with a flawed approach, and failed to achieve a satisfactory relationship. He then drew the erroneous conclusion that the reason for lower compliance among his tuberculosis patients, among other things, was their lack of a concept of prevention. He cited other authors who, like him, had drawn false conclusions,

I want to address this point, not only because of the error in his conclusions but primarily because his claim could be dangerous.

We get an example from Jansen about the difficulties to expect in forming a relationship if a doctor is not "patient-centered." Jansen wrote:

"It would be a little naive to think that as curative medicine has failed, preventive medicine now will be the panacea for resolving all the residual health problems. One has to realize that preventive medicine is not the most strategic way of introducing modern medicine in Africa. Alland (1970) who worked as an anthropologist in the Ivory Coast among the Abon recognized the communication problems associated with it: Preventive medicine is, in general, the most difficult concept to introduce. This is consistent with the hypothesis that much of what we would define as preventive medicine lies outside of indigenous theory. In many cases that westerners might define as rational preventive measures will be considered irrelevant by local people. In addition, since the introduction of rational preventive medical techniques must crosscut many areas of behavior, ongoing from such items as ritual and the formalities of social relationship to economic activity, they may be resisted because their acceptance would produce severe disruptions in areas of behavior which lie beyond medical theory and practice. The usual resistance to preventive medicine prompts us to reflect on indigenous practice and theories. The primary question which intrigues us is: Does African medicine in casu Bomvana medical practice know the preventive approach, or is this a pure western concept? The principal question is whether the discussed concepts of prevention have any affinity with each other. Prevention is based on etiology (Simpson, (1970), so western preventive measures have totally different foundations to the indigenous ones. The Xhosa concept of prevention is deeply rooted in their belief that the ancestors protect their well-being and that any disorder in tribal life is a sign of a disturbed cosmological balance. Indigenous healers dispense powerful means to restore this balance.

Prevention is aimed at propitiation the ancestors, hoping to receive their favors and protection. Psychologically it provides an armor which reassures tribesmen who feel surrounded by threatening dangers. The western preventive approach evolves more and more in the direction of control of nature and bears a manipulative character. It may interfere with certain physiological processes in our body (e.g. contraceptive pills) or may build up immunological mechanisms against pathogenic agents."

What Jansen reports about traditional preventive medicine among the Bomvana tribe applies in most respects to almost all of sub-Saharan Africa. But the question now is: does this mean that we lack a genuine concept of prevention?

One must distinguish between the implementation of preventive measures and the knowledge of their connection to the etiology of the diseases they aim to prevent. I am aware that prevention, by definition, includes etiology. Felix qui potuit rerum cognoscere causas (Virgil, Georgies II, 489). But how does this look in practice?

"Empiricism is based on the observation of facts, independent of any theory. Its place in medicine has been significant since the third millennium BCE and the development of archaic medicine. Even today, much of routine medical practice is based on it; it is empiricism that enables doctors to do more for the benefit of the patient than they understand."[xxvii]

Of course, the population in industrialized countries is closer to a preventive understanding rooted in etiology than in Africa, but nevertheless, the following is generally true:

"Empirical studies clearly show that patients' perceptions of illness (lay beliefs about the origins and nature of diseases) differ quite fundamentally from those of doctors (specialist beliefs about the etiology, pathogenesis, and nosology of diseases) (Boyle 1970)."

In Chapter VII of his book, Jansen provided many examples of "indigenous prevention" and could have seized the opportunity to build a bridge between "indigenous and Western prevention" had he not been fixated on his own system. He reports:

"Some Xhosa medicines are thought to have a preventive and protective power. Herbalists provide medicines for babies to apply on their fontanelle with the intention to seal it off for evil spirits as they might enter the child's body through this opening. A common preventive measure in use among the Bomvana is the use of a key worn on a necklace to prevent whooping cough in children. A similar situation has developed in Bomvanaland and increasing anxiety has enlarged the demand for protection against evil influence. It is disputable if one can say after Gelfand that "the African doctor, like the European one, appreciates the importance of the principle 'prevention is better than cure' for he too tries wherever possible to prevent disease. Apparently, there is similarity with western principles of prevention but by delving deeper, differences between the two systems become manifest. Prevention has to do with a certain time orientation, the effect of this medical action being in the remote future, e.g. poliomyelitis vaccination at a time without any threat of an epidemic."

Jansen became entangled in the minor differences here and completely lost sight of the most important aspect the common ground that he needed as a foundation for his "doctor-patient relationship."

Certainly, these words from Rogers are appropriate here:

'Most of what has been done in psychology can be compared to the early studies of primitive societies. The observer reported that primitive peoples ate absurd foods, conducted fantastic and meaningless ceremonies, and displayed behavior that was a mix of virtue and moral degeneration. What the observer failed to see was that they were observing from their own frame of reference and applying their own standards of judgment to the behavior of the primitives. We do nothing different in psychology when we speak of abnormal behavior,' 'delusion,' and so on. We fail to realize that we are judging the individual from our own or some general frame of reference, but the meaning of their behavior can only be understood if their behavior is seen as they themselves perceive it.

Just as the only way to understand another culture is by adopting the frame of reference of that culture, the same applies here. When that happens, the various meaningless and strange behaviors are recognized as part of a meaningful and purposeful activity."

This remark by Ulf Lind is also compelling:

"Active disease prevention is a common element across all cultures. *Naturally, it is adapted in each society to the respective concepts of various diseases. In the realm of natural causes of illness, people avoid, mitigate, or eliminate risks a very extensive activity in... 'I praise You, my God, and will bless You all the days of my life, because it has pleased You to anticipate for my healing that terrible day (of death and final judgment) by bringing the weakness You imposed on me, so that through it You already destroyed all things for me.*

...Let me rightly understand that the evils of the body are only a punishment and a full image of the shortcomings of the soul. But also, Lord, let them be the remedy against it, as You use the pains I feel to make me think of those things I did not feel in my soul, although it was entirely sick and covered with sores."

Thus, mysticism does not exclude the concept of "true" prevention. As mentioned earlier, Jansen claimed: "one has to realize that preventive medicine is not the most strategic way of introducing modern medicine in Africa." I disagree with this. I believe that preventive medicine or preventive measures "is the strategic way to introduce modern medicine in Africa." Just because the method and the ability to convince the population of the need for preventive medicine have not been successful, this does not necessarily mean that Africans do not have a concept of it. If a class has difficulty with mathematics, it does not prove that the students lack aptitude for mathematics it may be due to the teacher's poor pedagogy.

Jansen correctly recognized that a good relationship requires good contact.

"There is a bit more that should be said about contact with patients. Contact is an instructive word; the Latin root 'contactus' literally means: 'to go together in the same pace, the same rhythm' (Salomon, 1947). Much wisdom is concealed in this concept of contact in relation to our development aid programs. In history-taking we have to face the difference in general tempo between questioner and respondent. Probably we have often erred in talking with our Bomvana patients in that we drove our communication with them in too high a gear."

Here, I would like to add that this contact "marching in the same rhythm with the patient" is not only about the speed of the conversation but primarily involves an inner rhythm. That is, Contactus refers to an inner movement, stepping in sync and on the same level as the patient growing with the patient which aligns with Rogers' proposed prerequisites.

I want to give an example that shows how communication can be conducted on the same level with the patient, even when the concepts or underlying thoughts on the topic seem vastly different at first glance. Although the following case does not come directly from medicine, it still illustrates quite well what I mean.

A missionary wanted to tell the story of Susanna and Daniel from the Bible in the Old Testament to illustrate God's justice. However, the missionary knew from experience and the mistakes of other missionaries that one must take the needs and worldview of the population into account.

"When a young missionary has devoted twelve to eighteen months to studying the language, he then gathers himself for his first missionary sermon. The whole thing is carefully prepared, written out, and painstakingly memorized... He preaches! ... 'Do you understand what the European means?'

In most cases, the Black listeners understood the words, but these did not evoke any concepts; they did not create understandable images because the connection was missing. The young missionary had not yet attuned himself to the listeners, did not know their worldview, and had not yet learned to turn his academic knowledge into practical wisdom. On the other hand, the burning questions of his listeners, their specific needs, were still hidden from him. Because he had not yet learned to pay attention to their needs, the gift he brought was not recognized. Therefore, on the faces of the listeners, there was a secret rejection: 'I do not need your words.' Only when he succeeds in gaining insight and addressing the particular needs of the listeners does he work with success."

How did the missionary tell the story of Susanna and Daniel to be able to address the mindset of his listeners? Simply like this:

"A man sent ivory to the coast through his people to exchange for cattle. On the way back, the messengers talked among themselves, sold the cattle to the thieves, injured themselves, came back and said, 'Sir, the Masai attacked us on the road with overwhelming force, chased us off, and stole the cattle.' They pointed to their wounds. No chief knew what to do, until the matter was brought before Magiri. He had the young men brought in one by one and asked the first, 'At what time of day did the Masai come out and attack you? Where was the sun?' 'It was over there,' he said, pointing to the east, 'it was morning.' He was taken out and the second was brought in. 'At what time of day did the Masai come out and attack you? Where was the sun?' asked Magiri again. 'It was over there,' said the second one, pointing to the west, 'it was evening.' The two were placed in front of each other. In the confusion, they admitted their guilt and brought back the cattle. This story became famous throughout the land and is told under the title: The Cattle of Magiri."

The reader notices that the missionary has gained an overview: the goal is to tell the congregation about God's justice, His all-encompassing wisdom, as in the Bible. The terminology in the Bible is correctly acknowledged as a secondary matter and adapted to the mindset of the listeners.

However, if the missionary had been fixated on these little details, quoting them literally, the Africans would have had no interest in the story and might have fallen asleep. Certainly not because they do not possess the abstract concept of justice, but because the missionary skillfully and intelligently used the listeners' familiar background such as cattle, ivory, Masai, and the position of the sun. Now the communication is on the same level, and the result is fantastic: "The story became famous throughout the land."

Here is an example of how two different reference systems can be connected.

3. The Relationship of the Doctor to Primary Health Care

The doctor-patient relationship in Africa is additionally characterized by the lack of doctors. (See figure taken from "The Quest of Therapy in Lower Zaire" by J. M. Janzen, 1978).

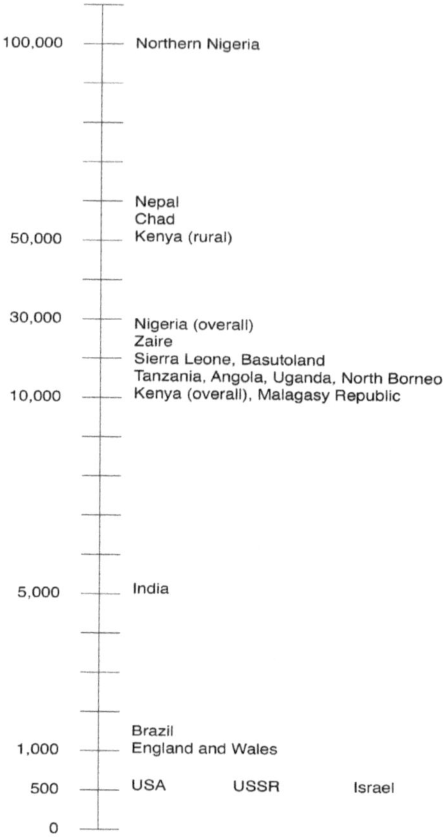

FIGURE 1. Inhabitants per medical doctor in several countries. Based on World Health Organization Records, from M. King. ed., Medical Care in Developing Countries (Nairobi, 1969).

Recently, the emphasis in Africa has increasingly been on primary health care and preventive measures. I believe this is justified.

"The new structures of the healthcare system are in line with the guidelines of the World Health Organization. It involves organizing primary healthcare'. Villages with up to 100,000 inhabitants are grouped into a 'circle'. At the head of each of these circles is supposed to be a doctor who oversees the activities of a team of nurses trained in a crash course. They are assisted by helpers who manage medications in the circles if any are available and the villagers must pay for them. These helpers, in turn, supervise the 'primary healthcare agents' in each village, whose role is simple but essential. They are responsible for distributing the medications and improving hygiene in the community. Maternity clinics are to be increased, and traditional midwives who assist in childbirth must be familiarized with basic medical rules.

The theory behind these efforts is appealing. There is no doubt that it is a way to alleviate the medical hardship of the indigenous population. However, the path from theory to practice is long. This practice has been started in the area around Bamako and in the southern parts of the country, where a doctor from Marseille, Dr. Hubert Balique, leads the new organization and faces immense difficulties. These difficulties are not just financial; tradition and the attitudes of the population are significant handicaps."

The doctor-patient relationship in such a situation can be crucial for the success or failure of these types of programs. Certainly, the long-term goal of primary healthcare should be to encourage self-help and a sense of responsibility for the health of the population.

The nurses, the medical staff, and the entire healthcare network responsible for providing medical care to the people in the country learn from the doctors not only how to administer injections but also how to interact with the population (even if they come from that population).

The doctor becomes the role model of a leader, and Rogers says:

"In the previous discussion of group-based leadership, it was repeatedly pointed out that some specific functions that the group-oriented leader brings to the group are gradually taken over by the group members. Group members become more empathetic in their relationships with others; they begin to listen more attentively to others; there is a growing understanding of the significance and intent of others' contributions.

In short, the members of a group whose leadership was essentially group-oriented seem to become more like the group-oriented leader in their attitudes and behaviors."

This means that the doctor first applies his doctor-patient relationship to his primary health workers, so that they can approach the population in the same way.

"The same dilemma arises at the beginning of the training of individuals in client-centered psychotherapy when they check whether their own fundamental attitudes toward people align with the 'technique' they are learning."

I believe that primary healthcare programs, or any health measures led by "non-patient-centered" doctors, will not achieve long-term success, and I fear there have been many such failures.

G. Walt and P.A. Smith from the London School of Hygiene and Tropical Medicine conducted a primary healthcare program in Mozambique.

"The forty-three students who participated in the study were the first group of técnicos de medicina (medical assistants) to be trained at the Health Sciences Institute, Maputo, Mozambique."

Initially, G. Walt and P.A. Smith asked the medicos técnicos to research some of the causes of illness as they are understood by the population.

Table 1. What causes disease?		
Factors relating transmission of disease	**Unrelated or 'magical' factors**	**Total**
21	20	41*

* 7 don't know

Table 2. What assistance was called for in case of mental illness?			
Hospital	**Curandeiro**	**Various**	**Total**
25	18	11	54

The specific etiology of illness was seldom known. The highest correct response (64%) was for the cause of diarrhea (flies or dirty water) and for the cause of malaria, 54% naming the mosquito (Gillies 1979). There was also some recognition that the effects of certain actions were linked with particular diseases - for example, tuberculosis was caught from going to work in the mines in South Africa. Thus, it could be said that with the common diseases there is often a commonsense explanation, although effect may be given as cause. The main objective of this study was to broaden the experience of the students and break away from the medical pattern of teaching, and only secondly to collect information. It was clear in the discussions that followed that it had been a valuable tool in sensitizing students to the strong cultural beliefs and attitudes towards sickness. They learned in practice the inadequacy of health education programs carried out with minimal regard for people's beliefs and material conditions, and the difficulties related to questionnaires and to analyzing data".

G. Walt and P.A. Smith have thus fundamentally recognized the necessity of teaching the "right" attitude to the trainees. Furthermore, such a method can be used to understand the reference system of the population. In discussions with the primary health workers, the doctor is not only informed about the reference system of the population with regard to a specific problem (e.g., the etiology of diarrhea, TB, etc.), but (after translating it into his own system) he is also able to pass on his attitude to the health workers with authenticity and empathy.

Such a method could often be used at the beginning of a health program. Suppose a doctor wants to introduce a child spacing program (contraception) in a village and start with "the pill." It would be wrong to simply explain quickly that the pill should be taken for three weeks, followed by a one-week break, and then give the women "the pill." In the long term, this could not only be unsuccessful but also harmful. It is well known through newspapers that in such programs, women sometimes ended up conceiving more children than before because they no longer saw the need for their traditional contraceptive methods, and they took the pill irregularly, either to save money or simply because the pill was not always available at the pharmacy.

"And the people in underdeveloped countries, with the exception of a small minority, are not able to afford medications whose price is disproportionate to their purchasing power, and in fact, is often significantly higher than in the West."

The doctor must first familiarize himself with the measures women use for child spacing. He should even approach it with a positive mindset, meaning he should expect that something is already being done in the population to address the problem. This can be formulated as a guideline: health programs that are to be accepted by the population must serve as a support or complement to the measures already in place and should never appear as "novelty goods" or as a new societal trend.

In our example of child spacing, it is widely known that, among other things, prolonged breastfeeding by African women has acted as a contraceptive. The doctor should calmly share this information with the women and health workers. He should tell them how beneficial breastfeeding (the skin-to-skin contact between mother and child) is for the child's psychological development. And as we know from statistics, childbirth and breastfeeding offer some protection against breast cancer for the mother.

"In the case of breast cancer, the risk of illness decreases with the number of previous births and the number of children that were breastfed."

This listing of positive aspects of certain actions that are already practiced by the population gives the people a sense of self-worth, and they approach the doctor with respect and an interest in cooperation.

Now I would like to say a few words about the importance of the doctor-patient relationship in collaboration with the governments of individual countries.

For example, how can a Primary Health Care program or education about hygiene, etc., succeed if the water supply and all public sanitation facilities are lacking?

E. Berger wrote:

"The decline in overall mortality and the resulting increase in life expectancy are demographic phenomena that occurred long before the major discoveries that established the scientific and societal status of modern medicine. The success of mankind in the fight against disease and death, which they represented, could therefore hardly be attributed to timely and accurate diagnosis or effective therapeutic methods in medicine. Rather, as the unanimous comments suggest, these successes were due to advances in the mastery of nature, particularly in the increase of agricultural, but also handicraft and later industrial production, improvements in water supply, and better hygiene practices. While these successes initially and predominantly benefited the socially privileged, they later and to a smaller extent benefited the poorer segments of the population as well.

Thus, the social prevention resulting from the development of productive forces is primarily responsible for the decline in mortalityin developed countries. Not only did the dangers of dying from malnutrition and undernutrition decrease social prevention, but it also simultaneously reduced the predisposition to infectious diseases and the ecological conditions for the spread of these diseases. The connection between social prevention and the reduction of typhus, malaria, and tuberculosis can serve as an exemplary case. Often several decades before the specific pathogens were discovered, the decline in mortality from many communicable diseases was already well underway."

Or as Prof. Dr. E. Seidler reports:

"Health, as it is now formulated, is the state for which the order of the state is designed and which is the condition for its functioning. In the industrial state, which is focused on work and performance, the illness of a member of society is primarily seen as a mere failure; while his illness makes him a private existence, his recovery brings him back into society. This was the starting point for a new form of interaction between the state and medical science, which led to many rightly celebrated health policy achievements."

The intense discussions, for example in Germany, about the proposal for a national vaccination law showed Bismarck the need to create a technical authority in matters of state health policy, one that could serve as a mediator between science and public health care.

This was done in 1874 with the founding of the Imperial Health Office, which later became the Imperial Health Department.

This reality was initially very fruitful and led to numerous social hygiene regulations and institutions with the force of law; I recall the laws regarding the handling of food, consumables, and utensils, the laws regarding the handling of wine, the legal appointment of food chemists, the establishment of an experimental and testing office for water supply and sewage disposal, and even the Imperial Contagion Law.

"The industrial countries have influenced Africa's progress so profoundly primarily because Africans themselves have failed to present an alternative model of progress rooted in their own traditions. For a long time, Africa reacted defensively to the model introduced by industrial society. The African attitude consisted either in retreating into traditions, some of which were otherworldly and focused on the past, or in a resigning and servile imitation of the work and life ethos of industrial countries.

This dualism permeated all layers of society. It caused divisions within the same region, tore apart families, and was the cause of individuals being torn between their enthusiasm for industrial society and their loyalty to traditional bonds.

All of this contributed to the destruction of the inherited village community and pushed the African - abandoned and helpless - into an unknown world."

Africa must assert its values

However, today more people believe that it is possible to break this vicious circle. Africa's only chance seems to lie in a philosophy that overcomes this infertile dualism. If development is to mean complete self-actualization for a people, it must be based on the assertion of the intellectual, moral, and aesthetic values that make up the collective essence of that people. Tradition and progress are not contradictory, but rather complementary ideas.

The only decisive question today is the choice between those indispensable cultural values that preserve the vital forces of the peoples and those values that must be abandoned because they hinder critical reflection and innovation. Similarly, a critical examination of the progressive elements offered by industrial societies is necessary to borrow only those that can adapt to our own societies and that we can develop with our own forces and for ourselves.

Further Reading

1. Cf. Len Holdstock, ***Indigenous Healing in South Africa and the Person-centered Approach of Carl Rogers***, In: Curare, Journal for Ethnomedicine and Transcultural Psychiatry, Vol. 4, 1981, pp. 31-46
2. Albert Schweitzer, ***Self-Reflections***, Munich, C.H. Beck Verlag, 1967, p. 103
3. Quoted in Sebastian Goeppert, ***Medical Psychology***, Volume 2, op. cit., p. 8
4. Leopold Senghor, ***The Word in Claudel and in Negro-Africans***, Dakar, Les nouvelles editions africaines, 1973, pp. 36-37
5. Leopold Senghor, ibid.
6. Cf. Len Holdstock, ***Indigenous Healing in South Africa and the Person-centered Approach of Carl Rogers***, op. cit., p. 32
7. Carl Rogers, ***The Power of Good***, Munich, Kindler Verlag, 1978, pp. 16 ff.
8. Paul Parin, ***The Contradiction in the Subject***, Ethnopsychoanalytic Studies, Frankfurt/M., Syndikat, 1978, pp. 86 ff.
9. Carl Rogers, ***The Client-Centered Therapy***, Munich, Kindler Taschenbiicher, 1972, p. 338
10. Leopold Senghor, ***Negritude and Humanism***, Düsseldorf/Köln, Eugen Diedrich Verlag, 1967, pp. 156 ff.
11. Cf. Carl Rogers, ***The Power of Good***, op. cit., p. 47
12. Cf. Carl Rogers, ***The Power of Good***, op. cit., pp. 21 ff.
13. Len Holdstock, ***Indigenous Healing in South Africa and the Person-centered Approach of Carl Rogers***, op. cit., p. 40
14. Cf. Carl Rogers, ***The Power of Good***, op. cit., p. 22
15. Sigmund Freud, ***On Dreams and Dream Interpretation***, Frankfurt/M., Fischer Taschenbuch, 1976, p. 12

16. Cf. Sigmund Freud, ***On Dreams and Dream Interpretation***, op. cit., pp. 14 ff.
17. Cf. Len Holdstock, ***Indigenous Healing in South Africa and the Person-centered Approach of Carl Rogers***, op. cit., pp. 33 ff.
18. Cf. Sigmund Freud, ***On Dreams and Dream Interpretation***, op. cit., p. 27
19. Cf. Carl Rogers, ***The Power of Good***, op. cit., p. 22
20. Sigmund Freud, ***Suggestion and its Healing Power***, Leipzig/ Vienna, Franz Deuticke Verlag, 1888, p. 177
21. Cf. Carl Rogers, ***The Client-Centered Therapy***, op. cit., p. 427
22. Gerhard Martius, ***Textbook of Obstetrics***, Stuttgart, Georg Thieme Verlag, 1981, p. 210
23. G. Jansen, ***The Doctor-Patient Relationship in an African Tribal Society***, Assen, Van Goncum & Comp. B.V., 1975, pp. 161 ff.
24. Cf. Sebastian Goeppert, ***Medical Psychology***, Vol. 2, op. cit., p. 172
25. Cf. G. Jansen, ***The Doctor-Patient Relationship in an African Tribal Society***, op. cit., pp. 162, 163
26. Carl Rogers, ***The Client-Centered Therapy***, op. cit., p. 427
27. Ulf Lind, ***Medicine among Indigenous Peoples***, Vol. 1, Historical Anthropology, in: Disease, Healing, and Medicine, ed. E. Seidler, H. Schippergers, and P. Umschuld, Freiburg/Munich, Karl Alber Verlag, 1978, pp. 54 ff.
28. Cf. Ulf Lind, ***Medicine among Indigenous Peoples***, op. cit., p. 77
29. Cf. Leopold Senghor, ***Negritude and Humanism***, op. cit., p. 44
30. Cf. G. Jansen, ***The Doctor-Patient Relationship in an African Tribal Society***, op. cit., p. 163
31. Karl E. Rotschuh, ***Concepts of Medicine in the Past and Present, Stuttgart***, Hippokrates Verlag, 1978, pp. 65 ff.
32. Cf. G. Jansen, ***The Doctor-Patient Relationship in an African Tribal Society***, op. cit., p. 77
33. J. Dannholz, ***In the Grip of Belief in Spirits***, Leipzig, Evangelische-Lutherische Missions Verlag, 1916, pp. 125 ff.
34. Cf. J. Dannholz, ***In the Grip of Belief in Spirits***, op. cit., p. 120
35. J. H., ***The Medical Misery in the Third World***, in: Medical Journal of Baden-Wurttemberg, ABW 8-81, 1981, p. 391
36. Cf. Carl Rogers, ***The Client-Centered Therapy***, op. cit., p. 329
37. Cf. Carl Rogers, ***The Client-Centered Therapy***, op. cit., p. 292
38. Cf. G. Walt, ***From the Classroom to the Community***, Teaching Primary Health Care Workers, in: London Journal of Tropical Medicine and Hygiene, Vol. 83, 1980, pp. 161 - 164
39. Ibid.

40. ***The Medical Misery in the Third World***, Medical Journal of Baden-Württemberg, Vol. 8, 1981, p. 392
41. W. Rotter, ***Textbook of Pathology***, Frankfurt/M., F. K. Schattauer Verlag, 1978, p. 217
42. E. Berger, ***Sick at the Crisis of Medicine***, Vienna, Europa Verlag, 1976, p. 146
43. Eduard Seidler, ***Western Modernity***, in: Disease, Healing, and Medicine, ed. H. Schippergers, ***E. Seidler, and P. Umschuld***, Freiburg/Munich, Karl Alber Verlag, 1978, p. 330
44. ***The Medical Misery in the Third World***, Medical Journal of Baden-Wurttemberg, Vol. 8, 1981, p. 392
45. Cf. Medical Journal, op. cit., p. 390
46. Cf. Carl Rogers, ***The Client-Centered Therapy***, op. cit., p. 422
47. Cf. Matomora K. S. Matomora, ***The Development of the Infrastructure in Medical and Health Services in Tanzania Since 1965***, op. cit., p. 27
48. Cf. Matomora K. S. Matomora, op. cit., p. 27
49. Cf. Amadou-Mahtar M'bow, ***Africa's Future***, The Integration of Tradition and Modernity, in: UNESCO Information Service of the German UNESCO Commission, Bonn, 26th Year, No. 7/8, 1979, pp. 7 ff.

Notes

[xxv] Matomora K. S. Matomora, The Development of the Infrastructure in Medical and Health Services in Tanzania Since 1965, University of Heidelberg, Dissertation, 1979, p. 47

[xxvi] Sebastian Goeppert, Medical Psychology, Volume 2, Rowohlt Taschenbuch Verlag, 1980, p. 123

[xxvii] Jean Delacreétaz, Medicine Between Two Barbarisms, Switzerland, Cahiers de la Renaissance Vaudoise, 1979, p. 54

SUMMARY

At the outset, I already indicated the intention I pursued when writing this paper. The doctor must understand the background and thought process of the African patient in order to foster mutual respect, which is the foundation for a healthy doctor-patient relationship.

In the preface, I introduced myself and my homeland for several reasons: Firstly, I wanted to emphasize that I personally engaged with the issue on-site. Secondly, I tried to show through the example of Mozambique how often the feelings and goals of the indigenous people were misunderstood by colonizers, some researchers, or other foreigners. This misinterpretation, along with political misconduct, inevitably led to health policy problems and disruptions in the doctor-patient relationship.

In the first chapter, the issue of anamnesis, or communication with the African patient, is described, and the importance of a good anamnesis for diagnosis, therapy, and compliance is emphasized.

Here, various possibilities for misinterpreting the patient's worldview during anamnesis by the doctor are discussed, and a real misinterpretation is shown through the case of M. J. Field.

Based on the reports by G. Jansen about his TB patients in Africa, I try to emphasize the importance of a good doctor-patient relationship for the success of therapy and cooperation with the patient.

In my opinion, the "failure" of many health programs in Africa is not primarily due to the traditional attitude of the patient, as is widely assumed; rather, I believe that approaches recognized in conventional medicine need to be adapted to African conditions (e.g., the attribution of the patient's role by the family with the support of the doctor's advice, not just by the doctor alone as in industrialized countries).

In the following section, I try to introduce the reader to the healing thought process of the African: the figure of the traditional healer has been at the center for generations. It is important for me to show colleagues that this topic — traditional medicine - cannot be ignored. Not only because every doctor in Africa is confronted with it, but also because the UN-WHO frequently recommends cooperation between modern and traditional medicine.

I share the opinion of Prof. Dr. Diesfeld that a "fusion" of the two systems can be dangerous for the patient if a serious and objective analysis and goal setting of these programs has not been examined and defined beforehand - as is often the case to this day.

I then list some achievements of the traditional healer, not only to show his significance before modern medicine in our culture but also to encourage the doctor to reflect. If a doctor is faced with a "foreign" custom, he should first consider whether this custom might pursue the same goals as conventional medicine in a different way. If so, he should support this custom and thereby create an opportunity for greater benefit and for building more trust with the patient.

I particularly warn against the use of psychotropic drugs. This is very important because our African reaction to illness involves a psychological emphasis, and the emotional complaints are at the forefront in almost every illness. The temptation for doctors to prescribe psychotropic drugs without thoroughly reviewing their indication is very great.

In the third chapter, I present some aspects of our understanding of life, death, childhood, and family in comparison to that of industrialized countries. I then attempt to address other important aspects of our worldview (e.g., Ntu = power = person, hence the word BANTU), which play a role in both healing and becoming ill.

I come to the conclusion that the African patient is not content merely with being treated, but also wants to be actively involved in the healing process, which has yet to be recognized by many doctors in Africa.

The phenomenon of "witchcraft" (bewitchment) is briefly discussed, and I examine whether there is any analogy to be found in European thought. I return to our African attribution of the patient's role by the family, where the doctor stands in the background as an expert advisor. I now explore the possible benefits of such an attitude, as well as the advantages of our African family structures, in the case of illnesses like heart attacks, cancer, etc.

I conclude that while the individuality and choice of the patient must be respected, the supportive role of the family and "environment," especially in chronic illnesses, including neoplasms, remains indispensable for the patient's recovery.

I believe that the psychological components of many illnesses are still underestimated in conventional medicine, and medical care in these cases still needs improvement.

Throughout the work, I highlight our "foreign" situations and ideas, attempting to explain them in the light of conventional medicine, and vice versa. This is not done to merge the two systems - they remain distinct but to seek a common basis that can serve as an approach for the doctor-patient relationship in Africa.

In the final chapter, I attempt to establish a connection between traditional African medicine and modern medicine. The focus here is on how a doctor can properly interpret the internal reference system of the African patient. I seek a model that is familiar to both the African patient and the doctor. I arrive at a similar conclusion as Len Holdstock, a personal friend and former collaborator of Carl Rogers, who also acknowledges that the approach of the traditional healer in conducting conversations has many similarities to Rogers' client-centered therapy.

I then compare the key points of Rogers' theory with the attitude of the traditional healer toward their patients. This is not only to confirm the similarities between the two but also to make the doctor aware of the expectations that the African patient brings to them. I use these similarities to take the next step: the "client-centered "therapy according to Rogers should serve as a model for building a good doctor-patient relationship. To this end, I provide examples of how, using this model, "the special medical history" or conversation with African patients can be conducted in practice.

The difficulties that G. Jansen faced with his tuberculosis patients in Africa, as outlined in the first chapter, now serve as a practical example to test the applicability of the model. At the same time, it becomes clear why Jansen's false assumptions (e.g., that Africans have no concept of prevention, etc.) could lead to dangerous health policies in Africa.

Last but not least, the doctor is encouraged to work closely with politicians. Aren't the many infectious diseases in Africa rather a reflection of the "medical and political diseases" (failures) at both national and international levels? Let's look at Europe. The eradication of many infectious diseases ran parallel, perhaps even as a consequence, with the increasing productivity and socioeconomic development of individual countries. Medicine in Africa should be an integration of traditional thinking with the positive examples and experiences from industrialized countries.

ABOUT THE BOOK

This book is about a series of my father's conversations with me in a poor Village, in Buzi, Mozambique, Africa. At the time of those conversations there were no storybooks for children.

My Dad used his genius to adapt his conversations to my age and as intriguing to my imagination as well as powerful, if not more powerful than the stories in the storybooks. They inspired me to use similar conversations for inspiration and encouragement of children of poor socio-economic status to become also a roadmap for success to a higher status. Those conversations allowed me, in spite of being born in a such poor village, to become a Board-certified physician by the American Board of Internal Medicine in addition to writing a Ph.D. dissertation with distinction of Magna Cum Laude

While in Medical School, I discovered a plaque, presumably a quotation attributed to E. Forest Witchcraft that read: "A hundred years from now, it will not matter what my bank account was, the sort of house I lived in, or the kind of car I drove, but that the world may be different because I was important in the life of a child."

This quotation inspired me to ask how can I elevate my father's conversation to an even higher level and include also to parents and children of higher socio-economic status? I decided to write the topic of my dissertation to be a blueprint for answering this question, as I show in the book

www.ingramcontent.com/pod-product-compliance
Lightning Source LLC
LaVergne TN
LVHW021737071126
851857LV00040B/1491
* 9 7 9 8 9 9 6 6 8 9 9 0 3 *